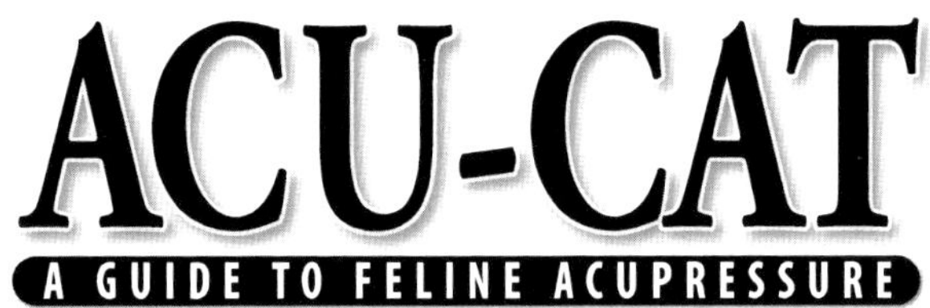

SECOND EDITION

Amy Snow
Nancy Zidonis

Foreword by
Michael Reed Gach

TALLGRASS
PUBLISHERS,
LLC

Castle Pines, CO

Tallgrass Publishers, LLC.
Castle Pines, Colorado
www.tallgasspublishers.com
tallgrass@animalacupressure.com

ISBN 978-1-936796-00-7
1. Cats 2. Feline Health 3. Complementary Veterinary Medicine
4. Animal Acupressure 5. Feline Health 6. Feline Acupressure
7. Feline Massage Therapy 8. Alternative Animal Healthcare
9. Traditional Chinese Medicine

SECOND EDITION • 2nd Printing

Library of Congress Cataloging-in-Publication Data

Book & Cover Design: Grant Dunmire, Attention Media Group,
Las Vegas, Nevada
Technical Editing: KimBauer, Lead Instructor,
Tallgrass Animal Acupressure Institute
Cover & Back Cover Photography: Cattie Coyle Photography,
www.ccoylephotography.com
Illustrations: Carla Stroh, Lusk, Wyoming
Anatomical Drawings: Janet Goldman-Merrill, San Pedro, California

Note: This book is intended as an informational guide. The approaches and techniques described herein are meant to complement and not be a substitute for professional veterinary care. They should not be used to treat any ailment, injury, or sudden behavior change without prior consultation with a qualified healthcare practitioner. It is recommended that cats receive regular visits with a holistic veterinarian.

Foreword

Perhaps the title of this feline acupressure book should be *ACU-PURRR.* I think that's a cat's content response when you stimulate their acupressure points. Cats love acupressure and are drawn to the points like a magnet when they are ready to receive. Your cat's feedback is instant; it's so rewarding and affirming to hear and feel your cat purr.

As the author of numerous acupressure books and founder of the Acupressure Institute in Berkeley, California, I have a deep passion for people learning acupressure in all its forms and applications. I was delighted when Amy Snow and Nancy Zidonis invited me to add to their Second Edition of *ACU-CAT: A Guide to Feline Acupressure.* I have been writing about and teaching acupressure for over 40 years. I am happy to support the launch of their new book. Their work has been instrumental in bringing the benefits of acupressure to animals and providing animal enthusiasts worldwide with a vehicle to better care for cats, dogs, and horses.

Cats understand the sensations and language of touch. The many cats I have worked on purred fully as I glided my hands along their meridian channels, stopping at acupressure points where the flow of blood and healing energy seem blocked. Cats are masters of their energetic needs. I believe that cats are much more aware of their energy flows than humans.

It is gratifying to watch cats preen themselves. Ever wondered why your cat will go over and over one particular spot on the inside of his or her hind leg? You know it must have been thoroughly clean many licks ago, but she continues to vigorously preen that spot. Well, your cat is probably giving herself an acupressure session. She knows her acupressure points because she can feel when blockages along the channels release and knows it feels good. You can tell by the way your cat moves and stretches her whole body – it feels more radiant and whole.

You may think you have domesticated your cat at home, however, they're not really tame – their vital energy is the same as cats in the wild. That's why they can become feral in a flash when left to fend for themselves. As cats live in houses and apartments, they become bored and lazy, which diminishes their vitality.

Like most animals, cats need to be invigorated to connect with their own vitality. By adding your touch, you can add just the right energetic boost to support your cat's health and wellbeing.

This Second Edition of *ACU-CAT* provides the instructional guidance people need to understand Traditional Chinese Medicine underpinnings of acupressure and its application for your very special cat.

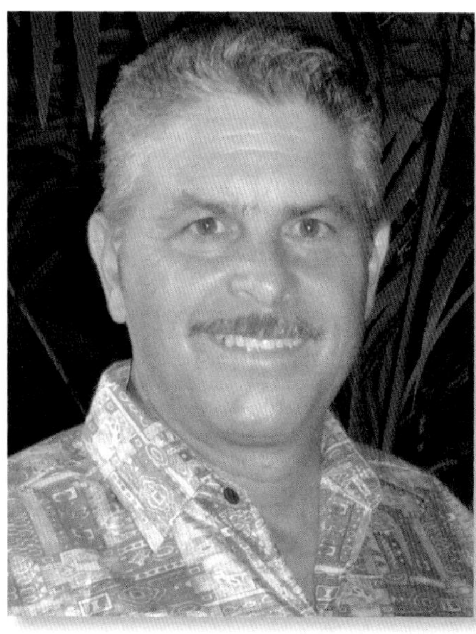

— Michael Reed Gach, Ph.D., author of *Acupressure's Potent Points* and *Acupressure for Emotional Healing*, fully illustrated self-healing of common complaints from A to Z. www.Acupressure.com

Contents

Foreword – Michael Reed Gach, Ph. D. iii

Introduction – Cats & Humans vii

Chapter One – Cats Will Be Cats 1

Chapter Two – Feline Acupressure & Traditional Chinese Medicine 9
- TCM – Thousands of Years of Healing
- Five Stems of Traditional Chinese Medicine
- Universal Laws and the Law of Integrity

Chapter Three – Traditional Chinese Medicine Theories 15
- The Theory of Chi
- Yin-Yang Theory
- Patterns of Harmony & Disharmony
- Five-Element Theory
- Zang Fu Theory

Chapter Four – Zang Fu Organs & Meridians 29
- Lung – Large Intestine
- Stomach – Spleen
- Heart – Small Intestine
- Bladder – Kidney
- Pericardium – Triple Heater
- Gall Bladder – Liver
- Conception Vessel & Governing Vessel

Reference: Cun Measurement 85

Chapter Five – Acupressure Points & Classification 87
- Acupoints
- Acupoint Classifications
  - Association Points
  - Alarm Points
  - Source Points
  - Master Points
  - Influential Points
  - Jing-Well Points

Chapter Six – Assessing Your Cat 103
- The Four Examinations
- Pulses
- Association and Alarm Points

Reference: Traditional Chinese Medicine List of Concepts 114

Chapter Seven – Feline Acupressure Session Protocol 115
- Phases of the Acupressure Session

- Opening Phase
  - Association Points
  - Alarm Points
- Point Work
  - Source Points
- Point Work Techniques
  - Thumb Technique
  - Two-Finger Technique
- Closing
- Post Session
- Cats are Cats – Short Acupressure Session

Chapter Eight – Feline Specific Conditions 139

- Local and Distal Acupoints
- Feline Aging Issues
  - General Aging Issues
  - Urinary Problems
- Arthritis
  - Worse with Cold
  - Worse in Wet Weather
  - Joints Exhibit Heat
- Behavior Issues
  - Aggression
  - Stress / Anxiety
  - Fear
  - Grief
  - Stress Reactions
- Gastrointestinal Disorders
  - Constipation / Diarrhea
  - Indigestion
  - Vomiting
- Immune System Strengthening
  - Immune System Issues
- Musculoskeletal Issues
  - Cervical / Neck Issues
  - Back Soreness
  - Hip Dysplasia
  - Shoulder Soreness
- Respiratory Conditions
  - General Lung Support
  - Bronchitis
  - Asthma
- Sensory Issues
  - Ear Infection
  - Hearing Loss
  - Visual Acuity
  - Conjunctivitis
- Skin Conditions
  - Dry, Itchy Skin
  - Allergic Reactions
- Spaying / Neutering
- Trauma
  - Heatstroke
  - Shock

Photographic Credits 184

Glossary 185

Bibliography 202

Index 204

Author Profiles 208

Introduction

Cats & Humans

Cats have become the most popular companion animal in the world. Their furry bodies and wily ways are so appealing. Their plaintive meows beckon us to satisfy their needs. Their independent nature makes them ideal companions for busy people. Cats fit in small apartments and large farms. They conform to being indoors or out of doors, romping and tromping. All in all, the domesticated feline is the perfect pet.

Cats have served as efficient mousers. The Egyptians discovered the cats' incredible talent for ridding grain storage bins of vermin. The felines, in turn, were attracted to human communities because of the ready source of prey. Our relationship with cats has been mutually beneficial for centuries.

During the medieval period, cats were feared because of their seemingly supernatural powers. Because of the cat's innate mysteriousness people identified them with the devil. By associating them with an evil force, people felt justified in viciously destroying thousands upon thousands of cats. Although the notion of cats being evil was pervasive at the time, many people protected cats knowing that their ability to control the rodent population aided humankind.

Cats have earned their keep for hundreds of years. As the 21st century unfolds, we have less need for the cat's impressive predatory instincts and a greater need for their soft purr, silky feel, and constant affection.

Today's feline is just as capable of survival without human intervention as they were in northern Africa hundreds of years ago.

However, by turning cats into companion animals we have imposed our world on them. This means we are depriving them of their natural environment where their keenly honed senses are necessary for survival. Cats have shown to adapt "just so much" to living with human (although, not to the extent dogs have adapted).

To live among us, cats experience stress. This stress is demonstrated by non-cat-like behavior, or by developing immune system diseases, or other health conditions. Acupressure offers a method of caring for your cat in a natural, loving way.

An ancient healing art based on Traditional Chinese Medicine, acupressure is noninvasive, and deceptively gentle. It can profoundly improve the health and well-being of humans and animals alike. Cats have shown to be extremely receptive to acupressure when they need it. Thousands of years of clinical observation have indicated that acupressure can enhance a cat's comfort, emotional stability, and overall health. Specifically, acupressure can:

- Build a cat's immune system
- Enhance mental clarity and calm
- Release endorphins necessary for reducing pain
- Strengthen muscles, tendons, joints, and bones
- Release natural cortisone to reduce swelling and inflammation
- Resolve injuries more readily by removing toxins and increasing blood supply, and
- Balance energy to optimize the body's natural ability to heal.

In recent times, modern medicine has begun to recognize the value of eastern healing modalities. Fortunately, we have the knowledge to make optimal use of both western and eastern approaches and techniques when caring for ourselves and our cats. Given the growing acceptance of the benefits provided by the ancient healing methods, more people are actively participating in their animal's well-being in this way.

However, acupressure is not a substitute for veterinary medical care. Rather, acupressure serves as a complement to medical services. When your cat is ill or injured seek appropriate medical attention from a qualified health-care practitioner. Acupressure serves as a complement to medical services.

Because cats are highly sensitive creatures and understand the language of touch, we invite you to explore the adventure of acupressure. Return your cat's loving purrs and willingness to be part of your life through this practice. Acu-Cat is a step-by-step guide into the realm of acupressure. As the techniques in this book give you and your cat access to health and well-being, it will also contribute to your mutual bond.

Chapter One

Cats Will Be Cats

Cats delight and mystify us. Domesticated cats are distinct from any other animal. We are attracted to their taunting manner, sublime expressions, and soft silky feel to the touch. Ever since cats decided to share their world with us, we've had mixed feelings about them.

The Ancient Egyptians considered these sleek, supple, vermin hunters to be deity. While they admired the cats' ability to perform their primary task of ridding the grain stores of pests, they also viewed the small North African cat as the connection between the world of darkness and daylight because of their nocturnal prowling. The Egyptians believed that the cat goddess, Bastet, would protect them from the dangers of the night when humans feel most vulnerable.

Thousands of years ago, cats were worshipped as a god. Cats have never forgotten this.

— Anonymous

Cats intrigued these ancient people. Their soft eyes contrasted with their relentless hunting nature. Their seemingly affectionate purring paradoxically opposed their unflappable stalking. When sleeping, cats appear to be the image of serenity, only to awaken to be treacherous killers. Rodents prove to be no match for the most benign felis domestica.

By the Middle Ages, these nocturnal, aloof, solitary creatures had lost favor with humans. Their behavior and appearance were interpreted as being evil and associated with the devil. In 1484, Pope Innocent decreed cats and cat lovers were subject to an Inquisition. Cats struck fear into the hearts of medieval Europeans because of the notion that cats had supernatural powers. No longer regarded as furry god-like charmers, they were hunted and destroyed by the thousands in the beginning of the Christian era.

Thankfully, some cats survived Pope Innocent's decree and went on to reproduce. Over the course of the next centuries, cats sailed the high seas as royal guests of captains and crews. They traveled to ports around the globe and were smuggled ashore to be sold for a pretty penny. In the New World, people valued cats so highly, they practically returned to being exalted as divinity. In the American West, the pioneers did all they could to acquire cats with kittens being sold for hundreds of dollars. With cats at their side, people recognized they could win the battle against vermin.

In this era, most people who share their homes with cats don't have the same need to rid their house of rats and mice as in yesteryear. In fact, most of us become squeamish when our seemingly docile, domesticated kitty brings home a half-dead mouse. We cannot deny that this is the nature of cats. In body and mind, they are still as wild as they were centuries ago.

Though barn cats and other working cats are still held in high esteem for their ratting skills, the predominant number of cats live as honored guests in urban and suburban homes. We overlook their gifts of shredded small animals, hairballs on our favorite rug, shrieks in mating season, and all the issues that go with cats living with us.

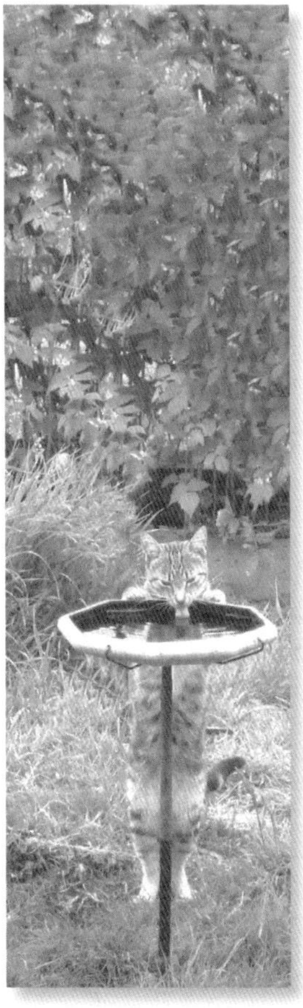

Adaptability and Stress

Living as our constant companions, cats have less stimulating lives than if they live on farms or in the wild. We ask them to adapt to our environment, causing them a great deal of stress. A city apartment presents little stimulation for a cat's hunting instinct. In urban settings, cats are apt to be hit by cars if left to their predatory nature. Suburban cats run the risk of absorbing toxic chemicals from fertilizers when dashing across a manicured lawn. They are also fed manufactured, grain-based foods that bear no resemblance to their natural diet.

With all of the trade-offs we offer, we expect our felines to be happy and healthy. Our devotion, cozy homes, relative safety, veterinary care, and abundance of food doesn't take the place of their nightly stalking of prey, munching on mice, and guarding their own territory. We think we're taking care of our cats – we are to a limited extent. We can't completely replicate an environment where a cat's natural way of being can be fully expressed.

To reduce the stress cats experience living with humans, people buy cat toys, cat stands, and cat window boxes. They even build screened-in extensions to their homes in an effort to keep their cat stimulated. People are turning to a raw food diet that comes closer to their original fare because cats are "protein obligates;" they must eat high-quality proteins.

All of these efforts are good. But there's another addition to your cat care regime that will greatly benefit his health and well-being. It is called acupressure.

Acupressure and Feline Energetics

Acupressure is an ancient healing art that has been used to support the physical and emotional health of animals for at least four-thousand years. Although some solitary animals prefer not to be touched, cats are highly attuned to acupressure. When your cat is in need of an acupressure session, he can cooperate and require little or no enticement.

After all, your cat intuitively knows more about the energetics of his body than you do. In general, cats are extremely sensitive, sensual beings, making them excellent candidates for acupressure. Once your cat trusts you're doing your best to keep him happy and healthy, he may demand an acupressure session when he is the least bit out of energetic balance.

Stevie, a middle-aged orange tiger, had been abused and neglected as a young cat. He developed a serious eye infection that went untreated. When we met Stevie, he was suffering from upper respiratory congestion and constant drainage from his eyes. He looked at the world through small slits and blinked his eyes quickly. His breathing was labored with a slight asthmatic wheeze at the end of each exhale. Stevie had received two rounds of antibiotics and seemed to respond well for a week or so, but then his congestion returned.

After Stevie's first two acupressure sessions, it became obvious his condition was improving. He began breathing normally and the swelling surrounding his eyes went down significantly, though there was still some minor drainage. Today, he energetically loves being the cat he's meant to be. Whenever he thinks someone might be willing to give him an acupressure session, he finds his way under that person's hand with amazing accuracy. He can guide someone's fingers to the exact acupressure points he needs to restore his energetic balance.

Clearly, acupressure gives you a therapeutic way to actively participate in your cat's health. By learning how to apply acupressure, you can create a close partnership with your cat, thus contributing years of quality companionship for both of you. The relationship you build with your cat will enhance his comfort, emotional stability, and overall health.

By combining the ancient eastern healing arts, current conventional medicine, your deep caring, and your loving good sense, you give something special and deeply caring to your cat. You expect your cat to join you in your hectic life, not realizing how stressful it can be for him. Acupressure gives you a means of reducing the level of stress your cat experiences.

When your cat is ill, injured, or demonstrating a behavior issue, consult your holistic veterinarian, animal behaviorist, or other healthcare professional. With many excellent resources available, it makes sense to turn to technological advancements. Acupressure complements other therapies and often alleviates the need for extreme treatments.

In practicing acupressure, as with any of the Traditional Chinese Medicine (TCM) disciplines, practitioners consider all aspects of the cat's life when assessing the cat's condition. You can't separate a cat's health from his environment, the food he eats, his routines, his general attitude, the amount of daily exercise he gets – even the look in his eyes. To understand how best to sustain your cat's well-being, the TCM practitioner has to consider a wide scope of attributes and lifestyle issues as well as the nature of this particular cat and felines as a species.

The Nature of Cats

Cats in the wild are nocturnal, predatory loners and extremely territorial. If we view feline behavior through the prism of territorial predation and the drive to perpetuate the species, even our domesticated cats' behaviors make sense. Their hours of incessant grooming and long daytime naps prepare them for their nightly hunting expeditions. You see, cats need to be extremely clean so they don't attract any unwanted attention. Neither their predators nor their prey should be able to smell them hiding or approaching. Plus, their fastidious grooming means fewer parasites and skin infections that could compromise their strength and survival.

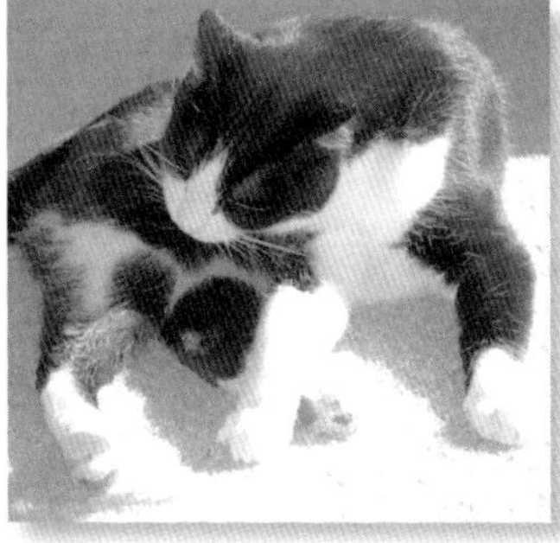

Nocturnal Predators

A cat's visual acuity is not particularly good. Cats have a limited ability to see detail but are quick to detect the slightest movement, even in low light. This makes their eyesight ideal for catching rodents that scurry and feed at night.

Practically every inch of a cat's body is a sensory organ. From the tips of his coarse whiskers to the end of his swishing tail, a cat detects a huge number of sensory cues. As evidence, the length of their whiskers matches the width of their bodies. If a cat wants to pass through a narrow space or a small hole, his whiskers immediately let him know if he will fit. Because rodents tend to hide in small, dark places, whiskers provide the cat with the necessary sensory information to avoid getting stuck in a place that doesn't allow him to move or leave.

Also, cats have extra sensory nerves on the back of their front legs. When catching prey, they use their front paws to clamp the small animal. Cats have to be able to feel the movement of that animal to know if it's alive or dead. If they let go of the small animal too soon and it's still alive, all the effort it took to stalk, chase, and capture is for naught.

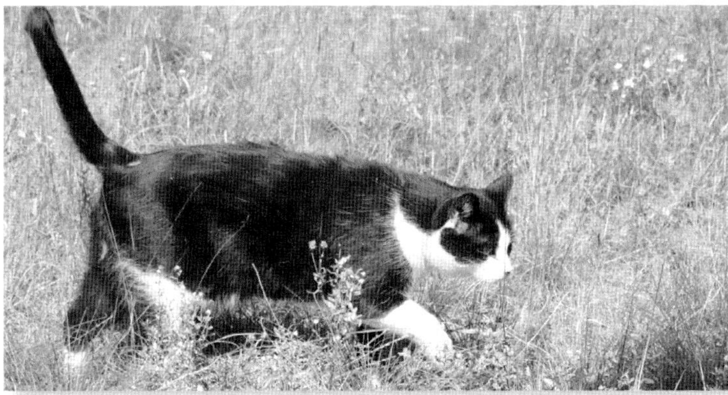

Although their sense of smell goes far beyond humans, cats don't use their olfactory senses predominantly to seek prey. Because mice and other rodents have a keen sense of hearing, they're alerted to the cat's presence if he were to sniff the air while stalking in the neighborhood.

Aside from the fact that the ears of most cats' are adorable and fascinating to watch, cats hear much more than humans do. They use their ears to communicate with other cats. In the wild, they provide visual and auditory cues. For example, when a cat flattens his ears, be smart enough to leave him alone - other cats do! Because most cats prefer not to fight, flattening the ears signals a good time to move on. If a cat needs to defend himself, flattening his ears actually protects them from being bitten or scratched.

A cat gathers auditory information with a minute twitch of his ears. Ears positioned on top of their heads like satellite dishes function as precise fact finders. Cats can instantly detect the location of a sound and know if it's moving and assess the size. They must use their senses for survival. Specifically, as cats catch prey, elude predators, they rely on their auditory perception to guide them through the perils of the night.

Solitary and Territorial

Because cats have to compete for scarce food resources, they carve out specific geographic territories and spend their waking hours patrolling and hunting within this domain. As kittens they grow and play together. But, as they approach adulthood, they challenge each other and go their separate ways.

Cat's territoriality gives rise to their need to mark the boundaries of their space. They have their own message system to let other cats know whether they're welcome or not. Urinating, spraying, and rubbing scent glands located on the sides of their mouths are telltale signs of a cat establishing or reinforcing boundaries. Cats emit odors ranging from very mild to extremely unpleasant.

Feline Domestication

Some people argue that our lovely pet cats are only marginally domesticated. They have a good point. Even while sharing our homes, cats still have their wily ways. They continue to defend their territories. They spray odoriferous signals when feeling threatened or a need to mark their territory. They prefer freshly killed meat to inert blobs or dry manufactured food. Face it; your cat still has all his basic instincts and habits.

As household pets, cats don't have to compete for food, and they have adapted to smaller territories. Many cats willingly share their space with other cats. Sometimes it takes a lot of convincing for an instinctively loner-type cat to accept another cat into the family. Two females brought up together seem to have the least resistance to living together in adulthood.

Because cats have been living with humans, many have shifted their lifestyles from nocturnal to diurnal. As a result, they spend their days hanging out on the window sill watching the world go by while making crackling sounds at the birds in the bushes. During the day, cats groom, sharpen their claws on scratching posts, and take cat-naps in sun puddles on the living room floor. When food is presented in a bowl, they have no incentive to sleep all day in preparation for a night of hunting.

Cats have proven to be adaptable, with each cat adapting differently. Handsome Spencer is content sleeping in his basket next to the fire place most of the day. He becomes a commanding tom in the neighborhood at night. Little Lilly, a delicate Siamese with a reverberating meow, might be too fearful and timid to venture outside at any time. George, a feisty apartment cat, bats small objects around the floor for amusement and exercise. And Sadie, an elegant Himalayan, can't imagine having another cat cross the threshold of her kingdom.

Ascribing Human Qualities to Cats

The point is, as distinct individuals, each cat has done his or her best to adapt to the environments we have created for them. We also have to be careful not to ascribe human terms and feelings when trying to interpret a cat's behavior. For instance, Toby urinates in a basket of fresh laundry. We might interpret this behavior as, "Oh, Toby is angry with us for leaving him alone" (or something like that). No, cats don't have ulterior motives. Toby might have urinated because of something stressful, but the odds are the laundry was in his territory and he needed to mark it to prove it was his territory. Tucker is not bringing you a gift when he drops a dead field mouse at your feet. He knows you will feed him so he does not have to consume the mouse for nourishment. A hunter by nature, Tucker is simply demonstrating his true nature.

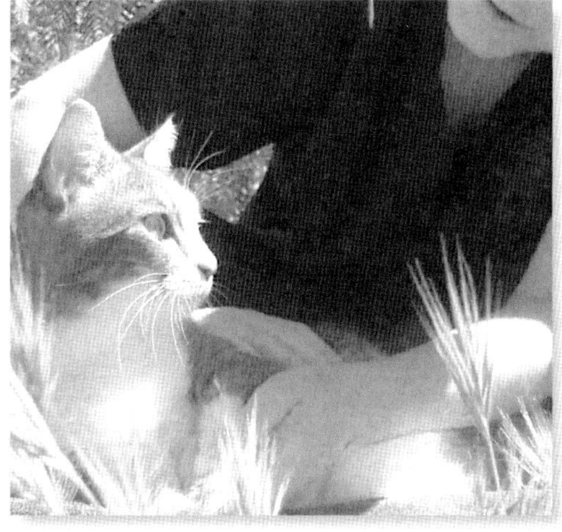

Domestication goes just so far with most cats. Think of how quickly and easily an abandoned feline becomes feral. Every cat is highly motivated to survive. Their survival instincts are incredibly powerful and they will do what it takes to eat, protect themselves, and reproduce. Once a cat is feral, it takes a lot of constant attention and food to reintroduce them to domestic life.

Cats' Wild Side

Don't expect human's to ever totally dominate the *felis domestica.* Cats will always have their own wild side and some behaviors can cause us stress. Yes, a hairball regurgitated on Aunt Susan's latest crocheting project can cause consternation. Claw marks on your favorite antique leather chair can bring tears to your eyes. And, running to the veterinarian because Darth defended his turf and now has a nasty abscess is no fun.

By associating with humans, cats have fallen prey to a host of illnesses and behavior quirks. They have become prone to diabetes, autoimmune disorders, allergies, skin problems, heart disease, obesity, urinary tract issues, kidney failure, and other health problems.

Cats are often traumatized by frightening things that happen in our urban and suburban environments. The rumbling of a garbage truck can strike fear into a cat's heart. A vacuum cleaner can have an equal effect to a cat's nervous system as that garbage truck. Fast-moving vehicles pose a serious danger. Certainly apartment dwellers know how destructive a stir-crazy cat can get without stimulation.

While we offer them food, protection, and healthcare, cats still have to contend with physical and psychological issues that compromise their health. Feline acupressure has shown to help cats acclimate more comfortably and healthfully to living with us. Cats and humans share something important; we need each other. This mutual need becomes our common denominator, fostering a bond that makes our destinies inseparable.

Cats contribute so much to our lives. What would we do without being able to pet their tantalizingly sleek, soft bodies'? Now, through the loving, healing touch of acupressure, we can return their gifts.

Chapter Two

Feline Acupressure & Traditional Chinese Medicine

Your cat is sensitive and attuned to his own life-force energy. If you watch your cat carefully groom himself, you will see he cleans and preens his entire body but also pays more attention to very specific small regions at different times. Chances are, his scratchy, rough tongue and paws are stimulating acupressure points and massaging the surface of his skin where it needs attention.

Did you know that when your cat eats grass, he is fully aware that his intestine needs clearing? In fact, he knows when he needs exercise, when to meditate, and when to sleep deeply. Your cat is highly connected to his physical and emotional needs. But as he has shifted from a nocturnal predatory lifestyle to a domesticated one, his existence has become more difficult and stressful.

Offering him acupressure sessions can help mitigate the stress he experiences living by our rules in the human environment. Once your cat trusts that you are assisting him in creating and maintaining a balanced flow of chi, he will show you how best to help him stay healthy.

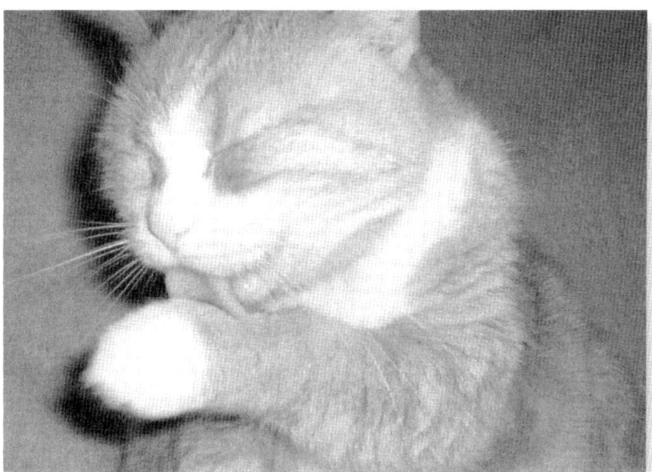

TCM—Thousands of Years of Healing

Acupressure connects you and your cat with thousands of years of natural healing.

This ancient healing discipline is one of the applied forms of Traditional Chinese Medicine (TCM). Understanding TCM takes years of in-depth study and practice. However, you can learn enough in a reasonable amount of time to have a profound effect on your cat's life.

Because Chinese medicine is a different mindset from conventional Western medicine, it takes study and time to learn Eastern concepts such as TCM. Yet studying it can be a rich, lyrical experience. Knowing more as you progress will enhance the effectiveness of your acupressure sessions with your cat.

Underlying Concepts

TCM treats the mind-body-spirit as a single entity. Within this mindset, the body – human or feline – is viewed as an intricate, interdependent system in which all aspects of internal life and the external environment intertwine. Supporting your cat's ability to exist healthfully within his environment is the goal.

Chinese medicine focuses on assisting the body to adjust to constant internal and environmental change.

TCM as it applies to animals developed as a preventive form of healthcare. It was used in ancient China to maintain the health of livestock – a valued resource in Chinese civilization. Thousands of years later, TCM is emerging as an important segment in the continuum of animal healthcare. Trained animal guardians and healthcare practitioners are offering cats, dogs, and horses the benefits of TCM through acupressure.

Five Stems of Traditional Chinese Medicine

In ancient China, TCM doctors known as "barefoot doctors" went from village to village throughout China practicing preventive care. If people in the community were healthy, the doctor would receive comfortable accommodations and lots of food. He'd be treated as an honored guest! However, when the people and the livestock in the community weren't healthy, the

doctor wouldn't be treated well. The rationale was simple: Why reward a doctor who was not keeping the community healthy?

The ancient Chinese recognized that everything is "medicine." In TCM, health is defined as an internal and external balance of nutrients and chi energy that allows the body to function properly. Said another way, Chinese medicine focuses on assisting the body to adjust to constant internal and environmental change. Consequently, five branches or stems were formed as a guide to achieving balance and health as change occurs.

The five stems are:

- Acupuncture
- Diet
- *Chi Gong* (Exercise technique)
- Herbal supplements
- Acupressure / Tui Na (Chinese Meridian Massage)

Acupuncture and acupressure are different applications of the same TCM principles. But because acupuncture is invasive, the thin needles used during an acupuncture treatment can only be applied by veterinarians trained in feline acupuncture and Traditional Chinese Medicine.

For diet, providing cat-appropriate food is absolutely essential to enliven a cat's energy; so is body movement through exercise or chi gong. Herbal supplements need to be prescribed by a trained veterinarian because they are ingested. However, acupressure can be safely offered to a cat by his guardian or a trained practitioner.

All mammals need to be touched. To enhance a cat's capacity to receive caring sensory stimulation and balance energy, cat guardians and practitioners turn to acupressure, or Tui Na. A cat's guardian can offer acupressure safely to their cat.

Remember, your cat wants to be healthy and sees no need to hold on to his hurts the way humans tend to do. When your cat requires energetic balancing, he can be quite demanding, so giving him acupressure will help him maintain his health and well-being. And the connection created while doing acupressure will gratify you both.

Universal Laws and the Law of Integrity

Traditional Chinese Medicine is made up of theories. The concepts underlying these theories are based on universal laws of nature. For instance, universal law says human beings and other animals are an integral part of nature. Our bodies are subject to the environment in which we live and must be adaptive enough to be healthy and balanced during the seasonal changes.

… the Law of Integrity states that when an imbalance is occurring internally, it will manifest externally.

Also inherent in Chinese medicine is that the living body is an integrated system. Specifically, the Law of Integrity states that when an imbalance is occurring internally, it will manifest externally. For example, when the Liver is not able to function properly, the whites of the eyes can appear yellow or jaundiced.

This concept of total body integration includes the emotions, which are part of how the body functions. Extreme anger often shows up as a red face, bulging eyes, and increased body heat. Because anger is related to the Liver, excessive anger can actually injure the Liver. Similarly, excessive grief can damage the Lung and lead to respiratory illnesses. These are only a few examples of how everything in the body is interrelated.

The Law of Integrity dictates that TCM practitioners must consider the entire being within its environment when treating an human or animal. This includes how they live each day, so lifestyle factors – exercise, work, rest, play, dietary habits, social activities, spiritual connection, mental engagement, etc. – must be factored into health assessments. The TCM practitioner asks seemingly strange questions such as "Which season does your cat enjoy most? Does your cat like to sleep near the fireplace or away from it in the winter?" Know that your answers help the practitioner sort out your cat's natural inclinations and environment preferences.

In summary, before grappling with the theories that constitute Traditional Chinese Medicine, you want to adopt the concept or mindset of the body being an integrated system subject to the Law of Integrity.

Key TCM Theories

Because basic TCM theories underlie acupressure, having a working knowledge of these theories helps you understand how acupressure works and how your sessions are affecting your cat.

The following chart gives you an overview of the essential TCM theories. Chapter Three addresses these theories in more depth.

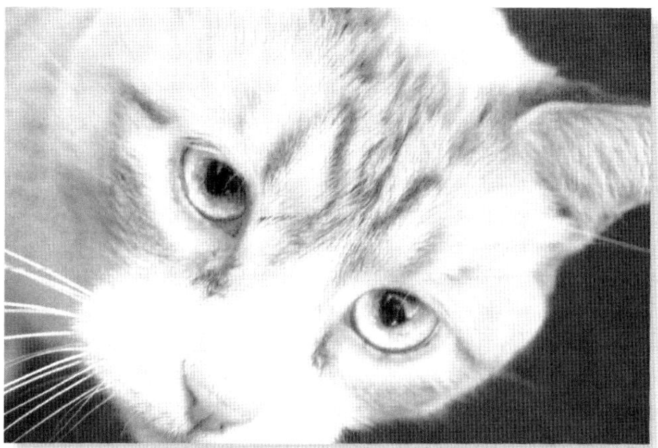

"If you are worthy of its affection, a cat will be your friend, but never your slave." —Theophile Gautier

Key Traditional Chinese Medicine Theories

Chi	Life-promoting force that is intrinsic to all living beings.
Yin / Yang	The two opposing yet complementary and interdependent aspects of chi that are in constant dynamic balance in living beings.
Zang-Fu Organs	Functions attributed to the internal organ systems.
Meridian	Channels or pathways that are extensions of the internal organs, along which chi and blood flow harmoniously to nourish the body.
Five-Element or Five Phases of Transformation	A conceptual framework representative of the natural phases of transformation and cycles of life and seasonal / environmental changes.

Chapter Three

Traditional Chinese Medicine Theories

Chinese medicine has evolved over centuries and was passed down through oral tradition before it became codified during the Warring States period (475-221 B.C.E.). The first known text, The Classic of Internal Medicine, or Neijing Suwen, is believed to be written by Huang Di, the Yellow Emperor.

In the huge country of China, communication from one part to another must have taken decades during ancient times. Yet, the theories and even the energetics of acupressure points (also call "acupoints") were, and are much the same today as they were centuries ago. Amazingly, this body of knowledge has been passed down in a cohesive and coherent way.

The Theory of Chi

The theory of chi differentiates Chinese medicine from all other forms of medicine and philosophies. It is based on thousands of years of keen observation beginning in primitive society and becoming increasingly refined and sophisticated.

When the ancient Chinese looked at the universe and life on earth, they realized there must be something that makes the difference between being alive and being dead. They called that living quality chi (also written qi or ki and pronounced "chee"). Ancient Chinese scholars were most interested in understanding the nature of life: What is that spark that enlivens the body? Their answer was chi, the life-promoting force that makes the difference between life and death. All living things embody chi.

Tai Ji Symbol

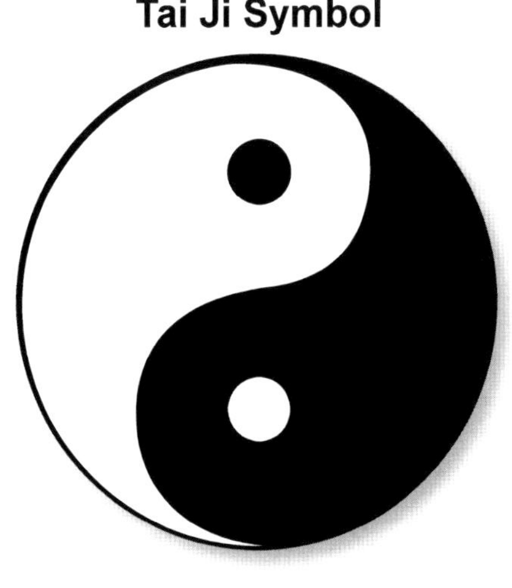

Yin-Yang

In its most basic expression, chi is the life-promoting energy that constantly flows along pathways throughout the body, nourishing the organs, tissues, and bones. This nourishment is necessary for the living body to function.

Without chi, nothing would move in the cat's body. Blood would stagnate and turn cold. No bodily functions would occur. Comparing a living cat to a cat that just died, the anatomy would be the same, but the spark of life that motivates and energizes a dead cat's body would be gone.

Chi is responsible for all of the vital functions of the body. To be able to differentiate physiological and emotional issues concerning the many roles chi plays in the body, the ancient Chinese ascribed specific functions to different types of chi.

For instance, three major types of chi are Source Chi, Defensive Chi, and Immune System Chi.

Source Chi, *Yuan Chi*, is the original chi a kitten inherits from the tom and queen (parents) that's stored in the Kidney. In TCM texts, this chi is often called Heavenly Chi or Prenatal Chi. Every kitten is born with a specific amount of original or source chi that dissipates as the animal grows, ages, and dies. It is responsible for the growth, development, reproduction, and proper functioning of the internal organs of the cat.

Kittens that come into this world through poor breeding or a sick, malnourished queen will have shorter life spans and will most likely fall prey to disease. But when the tom and queen are healthy, their kittens start life with a good amount of Source chi. Although Source chi cannot be replenished, it can be supported and sustained. It's up to you, as their guardian, to provide a healthy, balanced lifestyle throughout your cat's life.

Defensive Chi, *Wei Chi*, is the combination of the air chi of the lungs and chi derived from nutrients the cat processes. This combination of Lung chi and Nutrient chi creates Defensive chi that defends your cat's body from harmful external pathogens. This type of chi is also called Protective chi. The Lung organ system is responsible for sending Defensive chi out to the surface of the body. This way, cold, heat, and dampness can't penetrate the body and disrupt the harmonious flow of chi and blood that nourishes the internal organs and other body tissues.

Defensive chi relates to a strong immune system. Because of environmental pollution and the increasing presence of disease-causing contaminants, cats need to have strong Protective chi. Offering your cat an Immune System Strengthening acupressure session every five or six days helps build your cat's level of natural protection.

Because of environmental pollution and the increasing presence of disease-causing contaminants, cats need to have strong Protective chi.

Immune System Chi, *Zheng Chi*, is the cat's overall ability to ward off disease-causing internal and external pathogens (*Xie Chi*). *Zheng Chi* refers to the need to have the internal organs and the defensive chi functioning properly to resist pathogens. When your cat's immune system is strong, pathogens cannot invade his body and cause illness.

If your cat gets upset or stressed in any way, this immune system chi can become compromised. This in turn can lead to internal organs not receiving a harmonious flow of chi and blood. Lack of sufficient chi and blood can lead to the organ systems not functioning properly. When any organ system experiences a breakdown in chi, an imbalance occurs.

Although we can define the different functions of chi, we can't separate these functions; they must all work in concert to sustain life. However, we can identify different forms of chi to ascertain which type of chi is, or is not, working to the cat's advantage. For instance, if your cat experiences consistent nasal congestion, you know his immune system chi is not strong enough to resist cold pathogens. Indeed, they have already entered his body.

Yin-Yang Theory

Understanding yin and yang is the next important step in learning how chi functions based on TCM. Yin and yang are the two major aspects of chi. Yin is a form of energy that must balance yang, its opposite yet interdependent form of energy.

The ancient Chinese thoroughly and deeply understood the dialectic cycle of life. They could see that the crops would grow plentifully when they received hot summer sun during the day, the necessary portion of rain, and the right amount of cooling during the night. When it was dark, cold, and rainy for too many summer days, the crops didn't flourish. When

"The point where pathogenic factors invade the body is bound to be a place where chi is deficient."

— "Treatise on Fevers" from *Plain Questions*

there wasn't enough rain and the hot sun beat down on the crops on long summer days, crops couldn't grow vigorously. Clearly, growth and health depended entirely on the proper yin-yang balance of sun, heat, rain, and cool to create and nourish life on earth. Everything in nature must have a balance of day and night, heat and cool, dry and wet to thrive.

Nature of Yin and Yang

Yin and yang, the two dynamic forces that constitute chi, must be in balance for the natural environment and the living body to be healthy. Yin and yang are likened to the nature of fire and water in these ways:

Yang is like Fire	Yin is like Water
Hot	**Cold**
Active	**Slow**
Dry	**Wet**
Action is upward	**Action is downward**
Red (Light)	**Blue or Black (Dark)**
Consumes	**Nourishes**
Lacks density	**Has substance**

For your cat's body to thrive, yin and yang must be in dynamic balance. When he feels tired all the time and sleeps in sun pools on the floor, he might be experiencing more yin than yang energy as he seeks to warm himself. And when your cat dashes up and down the hallway like a maniac, he is expressing more yang than yin energy.

While yin is more nourishing than yang, yang is thought of as the active, moving aspect of chi. Circulation of blood requires yang energy while the nourishing quality of blood is yin in nature.

Yin and yang cannot exist without the other. If they separate, death occurs. Yin and yang are chi; they are one entity. When there's too much yin, there's less yang; it is said that yin has consumed yang. For example, yin is consuming yang when your cat has been out all night in frigid temperatures and arrives home feeling cold to the touch. In this case, the cold of yin is greater than the warmth of yang.

Because yin and yang are interdependent, the opposite happens, too. When yang is greater than yin, yin is consumed by yang. A high fever indicates yang overtaking yin.

Remember, the interdependence of yin and yang means they have to control each other so that the body can stay in dynamic balance.

When yin and yang are not controlling each other and maintaining a harmonious flow of chi and blood, your cat will show signs of ill health. Some blockage is impeding the natural flow of nourishment and energy. When this happens, you can read the indicators and know if it's an imbalance of yin or yang.

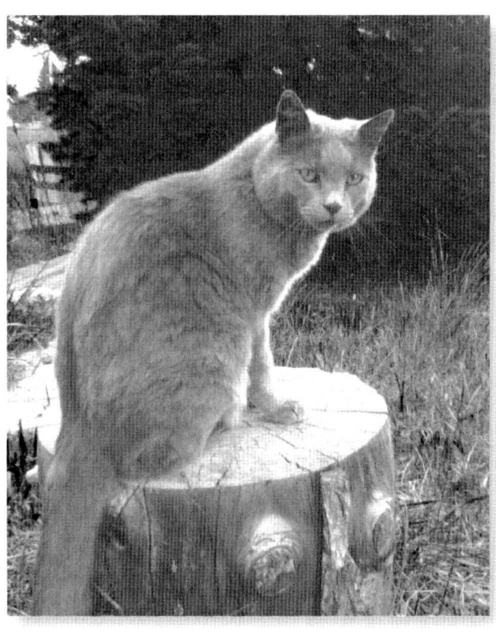

Blood is the mother of chi.
Chi is the commander of blood.

On The Body

Yin	Yang
Foot	Head
Chest / Abdomen	Spine / Back
Female	Male
Interior of body	Surface of body
Older	Younger

Temperament

Yin	Yang
Withdrawn	Outgoing
Timid	Aggressive
Quiet	Loud
Low activity	Highly active
Calm	Anxious
Relaxed	Energetic
Gentle	Rough

On Earth

Yin	Yang
Water	Fire
Cold	Hot
Wet	Dry
Earth	Heaven
Moon	Sun
Night	Day
Winter	Summer
Below	Above
Dark	Light

Patterns of Harmony and Disharmony

When yin and yang are balanced, the internal organ systems can function properly because they are receiving chi, blood, and other vital substances necessary for healthy activity. Consequently, your cat's body and mind can function within his climatic and social environment. A healthy cat is friendly, energetic, and confident, with bright eyes, shiny coat, white teeth, light pink gums, and a natural tongue with pulses that are smooth, strong, and firm. The cat exudes health and health is considered a pattern of harmony.

Also, the body needs hot and cold, wet and dry. Too much of one or too little of another leads to an imbalance of yin and yang. If your cat has a fever, this is more of a yang than a yin indicator because it is hot. We often phrase this type of imbalance as a Yang Pattern of Disharmony.

Other yang patterns of disharmony include dehydration, constipation, loss of weight, hyperactivity, inflammation, anger, fast pulse, and red tongue. Notice, all of these are heat related. After it rains, puddles form. The sun comes out and the puddles evaporate. Too much heat leads to dehydration.

In the body, constipation indicates a lack of moisture in the feces. When a cat experiences a loss of weight, he is losing substance and fluids. Hyperactivity and anger indicate the cat is expending heat energy. These forms of imbalances are also referred to as Heat Syndromes.

Yin patterns of disharmony are characterized by lethargy, being overly-hydrated, edema, weakness, stumbling, low body temperature, not healing, poor digestion, depression, pale tongue, slow pulse, and any type of hypo-functioning. These conditions are all associated with the animal experiencing too much cold and wet like the nature of water. Indicators that are yin in nature are often referred to as Cold Syndromes.

Yin in excess injures yang; yang in excess injures yin.
A preponderance of yang creates manifestations of heat;
a preponderance of yin brings on cold manifestations.

— "Treatise on the Correspondence between Man and the Universe" in *Plain Questions*

Summary of Yin-Yang Theory

The Yin-Yang Theory provides a point of access for dealing with disease. When the animal is healthy, yin and yang are in balance and chi performs all the roles that maintain health. However, when there's an imbalance of yin and yang, chi and blood cannot warm and nourish the cat or protect him from pathogens. Common sense dictates the value of maintaining a balance of yin and yang by supporting a healthy lifestyle.

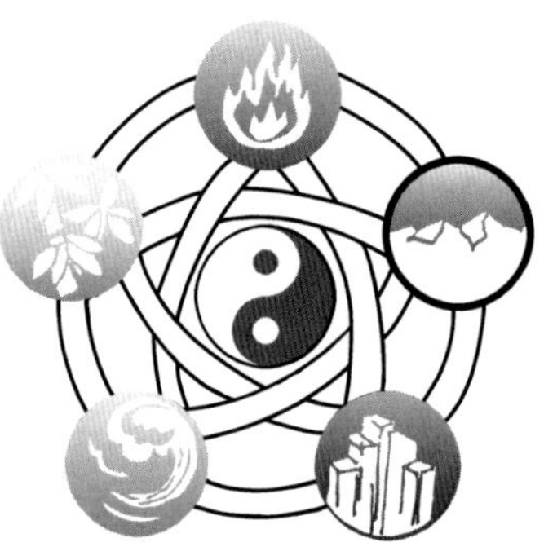

In its wisdom, Chinese medicine focuses on prevention of illness. By offering your cat acupressure sessions, you can support his immune system consistently by stimulating the movement of chi and blood throughout his body, thus maintaining his yin-yang balance.

Five-Element Theory

The Five-Element Theory is a construct derived from Taoist philosophy. This theory, with the Yin-Yang Theory, represents the core of Traditional Chinese Medicine.

In Chinese, the Five Elements are called *Wu Zing. Wu* means five while *Zing* can be translated as "movement, change, transition, transformation, or process." Thus, the original intent was to refer to the Five Phases of Transition or the Five Phases of Transformation. In the West, it is common to refer to these five phases as "elements" because they are identified as five constituents of nature: Wood, Fire, Earth, Metal, and Water.

The Five-Element Theory created a logical model for life and the natural environment. The ancient Chinese studied the universe and saw that everything is related to everything else. Crops cannot grow without the balance of sun, water, and cool nights. Humans and animals cannot live healthfully without nourishment derived from rice and other grains that grow on earth. Thus, the Five-Element Theory is based on a profound understanding of the interrelatedness of heaven and earth. All natural phenomena must be in a dynamic state of balance for the health of all living things to exist. This includes the earth and all creatures.

The ancient Chinese use the term "elements" to represent a host of properties within which each of the five natural constituents can be identified. Each element is a symbol or metaphor representing attributes that indicate the seasonal cycle, life cycle, direction of energy, relative body tissues, emotions, internal organ systems, and many more correspondences.

木 **Wood** represents birth, rebirth, spring, and upward, exuberant energy. Wood is associated with tendons and ligaments of the body because, like young saplings, they have to be flexible and strong enough to bend in the winds of spring. Liver and Gall Bladder are the organ systems associated with Wood because, after thousands of years of applying TCM, we know they directly affect the health of the tendons and ligaments. The emotion related to Wood is anger. (Think of liver bile that suggests the emotion of anger.)

火 **Fire** energy is expansive and rises. The season of Fire is summer, the hottest time of the annual cycle, the season of the greatest growth. Growth is considered the life cycle stage of Fire. Because it is the hottest color, the color associated with Fire is red. The main yin organ system for Fire is the Heart, Monarch of the Body, responsible for the fair apportionment and circulation of warmth and nourishment of the body. The emotions of Fire is joy. (Think of how joy affects the Heart function.)

土 **Earth** energy is centered in the way the Stomach and Spleen are centered in the body. The Earth produces food to nourish the body. The maturing of crops in late summer corresponds with the energy of Earth. The Spleen and Stomach are responsible for creating bio-absorbable nutrients. The muscles and four limbs require nourishment to be strong. Worry is the emotion of Earth. (Think about how worry can greatly affect digestion and feeling centered or grounded.)

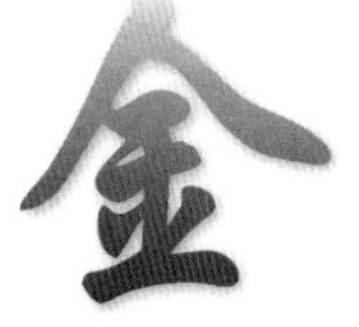

Metal energy is contracting, like the gathering-in of the harvest in autumn. The Lung and Large Intestine are the Metal organ systems. The Lung gathers chi from the air and the Intestine collects waste matter. The emotion of Metal is grief. (Think how the walls of the Lungs tighten during times of grief or sorrow – the lung tissue actually thickens.)

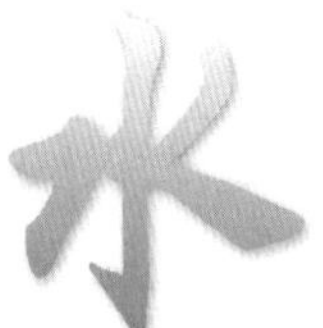

Water is related to the cold of winter when conserving energy is necessary. Human and animal energy turns inward. Cats love to curl up in a warm place during dark, cold winter days. This element is related to old age and the end of a cycle. The Kidney and Bladder organ systems correspond with Water because they are involved with the water metabolism of the body. Kidney governs bones, which make up the core strength of the body. Water is related to will power, which also reflects core strength. The emotion of Water is fear. (Think how cats can urinate or spray when fearful)

The Five-Element Theory provides a tool for understanding the natural flow of life and energy. Many practitioners use it for identifying patterns in animals. If a cat seems angry, his gait is stiff, and he avoids wind especially in the spring—all indicators suggest a Wood Pattern of Disharmony. By comparison, a cat with a Metal Pattern of Disharmony could exhibit lung and nasal congestion in the autumn.

Take time to meditate on the Correspondence Chart for the Elements. As you do, suspend your Western beliefs and be open to the lyrical, metaphoric qualities of the Five-Element Theory.

Zang-Fu Theory

The ancient Chinese wanted to understand how the body functions as a whole rather than isolating its parts. They knew everything in the living body was intricately interrelated. Hence, the Traditional Chinese Medicine view of the internal organs, called in Chinese zang-fu organs, differs significantly from conventional Western medicine view. The organs have the same names in TCM as in Western medicine except that references to an

FIVE PHASES OF TRANSFORMATION CORRESPONDENCE CHART

	METAL	WATER	WOOD	FIRE	EARTH
ENERGY	Contracting	Conserving	Generative	Expansive	Stabilizing
YIN-YANG PHASE	New Yin	Full Yin	New Yang	Full Yang	Yin-Yang Balance
TRANSITION / LIFE CYCLE	Harvest / Middle Age	Storage / Old Age to Death	Birth	Creation / Growth	Maturity
SEASON	Fall	Winter	Spring	Summer	Late Summer
CLIMATE	Dry/Wind	Cold	Windy	Hot	Wet/Humid
DIRECTION	West	North	East	South	Center
COLOR	White	Blue	Green	Red	Yellow
EMOTION	Grief	Fear	Anger	Joy	Sympathy/Worry
SENSORY ORIFICE	Nose	Genitals/ Ears	Eyes	Tongue	Mouth
SMELL	Rotten	Putrid	Rank	Burning	Fragrant/Sweet
GOVERNED PART OF BODY	Skin & Body Hair	Bones & Marrow	Tendons & Ligaments	Vascular System	Muscles & Lymph
MERIDIANS	Lung & Large Intestine	Kidney & Bladder	Liver & Gall Bladder	Heart & Sm Intestine Pericardium & Triple Heater	Spleen & Stomach

organ includes the entire system – that is the organ itself, its meridian, and all of the functions it performs.

Note: Any discussion of an organ in this book refers to the complete organ system. To signify a system, the first letter is capitalized (e.g., Liver refers to the whole liver system, not just the organ itself). Again, an organ system includes the organ and its related meridian or energetic pathway along with its functional and energetic activities.

Organ Systems

According to TCM, each organ anchors a multi-functional system. All the systems represent a host of attributes such as an emotion, direction of chi flow, sensory orifice, type of body fluid, bodily tissues it controls, creation and storage of vital substance, odor, taste, color, time of day and year for optimal chi flow, and even further levels of detail.

Many associated aspects of an organ system may seem esoteric, but by thinking about the Lung system related to grief, for example, you can physically experience it as real. Think about the cat you might have recently lost and take a deep breath. How does it feel? What you experience leaves no doubt that grief leads to physiologic changes in your lungs!

If an animal or human couldn't move on from grieving, a persistent constriction could result in respiratory disease due to stagnation of fluids in the Lung. It could also lead to other breakdowns in the body's immune system. Clearly, nothing is isolated. An inability of one system to perform its role within the body can present a pathological progression of indicators leading to a pattern of disharmony.

Studying the zang-fu organs gives you excellent access to how Eastern pathology is applied. Developed through thousands of years of observation and practical clinical experience, it describes the functions of the zang-fu organs and their energetic channels as a system. It further describes the relationships among the zang-fu organs as well as their effect on the body.

Zang-Fu Organs

Zang refers to the core internal organs, the yin organs. Most texts identify five zang organs: Lung, Heart, Spleen, Liver, and Kidney. However, some also include the Pericardium, the sac surrounding and protecting the Heart, thus making it six zang organs.

The zang organs create and store vital substances, including chi, blood, essence, body fluids, and shen (consciousness/spirit). The zang organs, hidden deep in the trunk of the body, are solid in form and nature.

Zang / Yin		Fu / Yang
Lung	&	Large Intestine
Spleen	&	Stomach
Heart	&	Small Intestine
Kidney	&	Bladder
Pericardium*	&	Triple Heater
Liver	&	Gall Bladder

* Some texts include the Pericardium as a yin organ; many do not. The zang-fu organs are typically presented as five zang organs and six fu organs. However, the Pericardium meridian is considered as significant in its function as any other meridian.

The fu organs are the next layer out from the core zang organs. These organs are yang in nature because their role is to transport substances such as food, water, and waste. These six organs tend to be hollow and tubular in form: Large Intestine, Stomach, Small Intestine, Bladder, Gall Bladder, and Triple Heater. (Chapter Four features a more detailed discussion of each organ.)

The zang-fu organs have identifiable relationships with each other. The most evident is their paired relationships with yin and yang organ systems paired like husband and wife or like sisters. The energy of one can balance the energy of the other because they are internally and externally related. For instance, the Lung is the yin organ system related to the Large Intestine, which is the yang organ system.

Chi, yin-yang, zang-fu, and the five-element theories are essential to Traditional Chinese Medicine. The more you know the more effective your acupressure sessions with your cat will be.

Chapter Four takes you another step toward putting theory into practice.

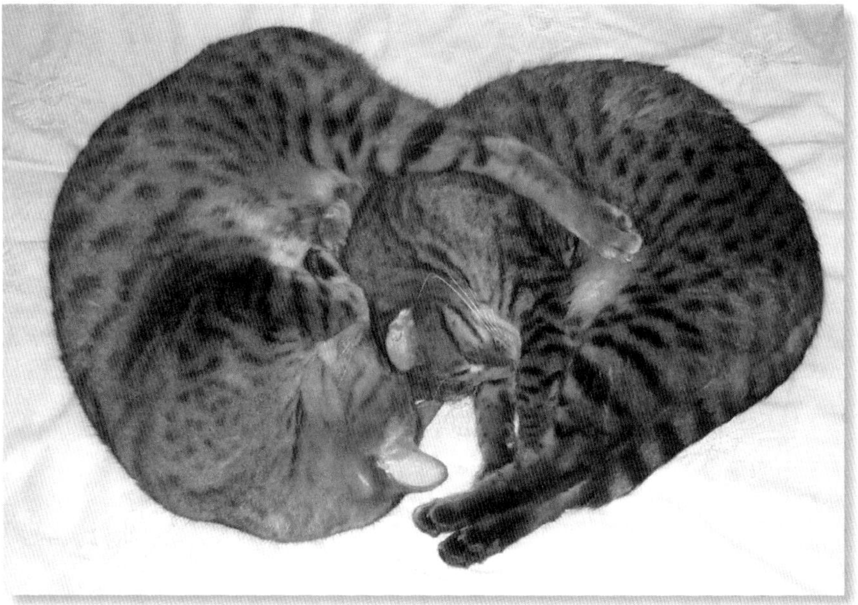

"Cats are rather delicate creatures and they are subject to a good many ailments, but I never heard of one who suffered from insomnia." — Joseph Wood Krutch

Chapter Four

Zang-Fu Organs & Meridians

Cats might be the most connected to their own energetics of all domesticated animals. They seem to be aware of the energetic pathways, or channels, also called meridians that flow throughout their bodies.

When watching cats groom themselves, you see they often lick and scrub specific locations where there are known acupoints. Cats carefully lick down the outside of one front leg along a meridian called the Large Intestine meridian. How do they know Chinese medicine? Most people don't! But now it is time for you to get up to speed with your cat.

Studying the *zang-fu* organs and their meridians is the basis of Eastern pathology. Each of the internal organs has its own meridian; the two together constitute an entire organ system. For example, the Heart organ along with the Heart meridian is considered a physical and energetic unit.

Meridians are internally and externally connected to the organ for which they're named. The organs are internal while the connected meridians are considered superficial because they run just under a cat's skin. In acupressure, you want to manage an imbalance at the meridian level before it penetrates deeply into your cat's body and affects the organ itself.

The Lung System and Other Examples

Let's look at one organ system to understand how acupressure works. The Lung meridian communicates with the Lung organ internally and extends the energetic functions of the Lung organ to the surface of the body. You can access the functional energetics of the Lung by working with the pools of energy, known as "acupoints," located along the Lung meridian. During an acupressure session, you can stimulate these acupoints to resolve an imbalance within the Lung organ or along the Lung meridian.

If a cat presents with raspy breathing and tires easily, you can apply pressure to acupoints along the Lung meridian, such as Lung 7. Thus, the process of balancing the Lung chi begins. By stimulating an acupoint, you are influencing the flow of blood and chi along the Lung meridian affecting the Lung organ as well.

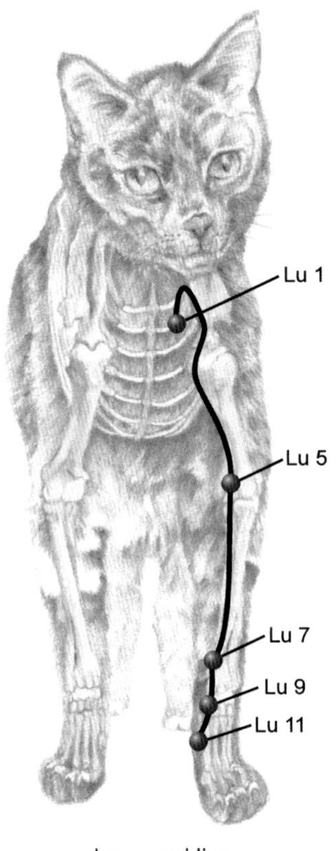

Lung meridian

In another example, say a cat sustained an injury to his carpus, or wrist. You could also use acupoints along the Lung meridian to help increase the flow of chi and blood to the area. Because the Lung meridian runs through the cat's wrist, doing this enhances the healing process. Remember, acupoints along the meridians serve to manage imbalances related to the zang-fu organ system as well as address trauma or other issues that occur along the physical pathway of the meridian.

Knowing the functions and energetics of the zang-fu organ systems is absolutely essential to being able to assess your cat's Pattern of Disharmony and helping resolve the condition. Each organ system has its own associated correspondences that provide indicators of balance or imbalance.

Because of the Law of Integrity (it says what happens internally will manifest externally), you can see internal organ and meridian imbalances. From there, you know how to interpret the imbalances by learning the functions and energetics of each zang-fu organ system. This is the key to Eastern pathology.

For example, the Lung is not balanced when your cat exhibits respiratory issues. (Remember, the Lung governs respiration.) When you see a discharge from your cat's nose, you know he has an imbalance in the Lung organ system (the orifice of the Lung is the nose and the fluid of the Lung is mucous). Body tissues related to the Lung are skin and skin hair, which means when your cat's coat appears and feels dry and his skin is flaky, you know the Lung organ system is not performing its job of supplying sufficient blood to the skin and body hair to sustain moisture. These external indicators show that the Lung is not properly balanced.

When considering the indicators the cat is exhibiting, you see a Pattern of Disharmony emerge and can figure out which organ system is not balanced. However, a number of clinical signs may present a complicated picture, making the assessment confusing. For simplicity sake, focus on the most obvious indicators—those that are most obvious or debilitating.

In conventional veterinary medicine, a cat that has an obstructed airway receives emergency care before the cat with a broken limb. In TCM, the lungs are regarded as vital, too. In Chinese medicine, the Lung stores the vital substance of chi related to the breath. Lung chi is an extremely vital substance. No breath, no life.

Meridians Link the Entire System

All of the organ systems are mutually interdependent. The meridians link the entire system to create a single network throughout your cat's body. If an organ were to fail, the entire network would fail. The network makes up a constant mutual support system, each organ performing its role within the system for the health of the organic whole.

Because the five zang, or yin, organs store the vital substances and are located in the deepest layer of the body, they can be regarded as the most vital organ systems. Imbalances in the zang organs are usually addressed first in an acupressure session. Imbalances within the fu, or yang, organs also need to be addressed. However, they can be seen as secondary unless there's an intestinal impaction, trauma, or other obvious emergency care needed.

The rest of this chapter lists the correspondences for the zang-fu organs and their related meridians. It includes charts and photographs depicting the flow of the meridians, along with the key acupoints for each meridian.

Abbreviation Legend

Lung – **Lu**
Large Intestine – **LI**
Spleen – **Sp**
Stomach – **St**
Heart – **Ht**
Small Intestine – **SI**
Kidney – **Ki**
Bladder – **Bl**
Pericardium – **Pe**
Triple Heater – **TH**
Gall Bladder – **GB**
Liver – **Liv**

All emergency care requires immediate veterinary attention.

Lung
Foreleg *Taiyin* / Greater Yin
Master of the Pulse

The very first independent act a kitten makes is to take his first breath and from that instant on, the Lung is in charge of his pulse. Lung, *Fei* in Chinese, is responsible for respiration and the tissues associated with the Lung. These tissues include skin and skin hair which also "breathes" and removes toxins from the body. The Lung is known as the intermediary organ between the body and the environment and as such is the most vulnerable of the organs to external pathogens. The Lung is the paired organ system with the yang Large Intestine.

Functions & Attributes

- Governs respiration
- Governs and stores chi / vitality
- Controls the channels and blood vessels
- Controls dispersing and descending of chi
- Forms Zong / Chest chi
- Circulates Wei / Defensive chi
- Regulates water passages
- Controls the skin and coat
- Manifests in the skin and coat
- Sensory orifice is the nose
- Fluid is mucous
- Emotion is grief or sadness
- Belongs to the Metal Element
- Optimal flow of Chi 3 – 5 AM

Health Issues

- Respiratory conditions
- Limited neck and shoulder mobility
- Lymphatic circulation
- Sensitivity to climate
- Skin problems / lackluster coat
- Poor immune system
- Allergies

Emotional Issues

- Chronic or long-term grief
- Compulsive behaviors
- Indifference or aloofness
- Stubbornness

Location and Flow of the Lung Meridian

The Lung meridian begins internally and surfaces in the hollow of the chest, where it meets the medial side of the forelimb in the pectoral muscle. This point is known as Lu 1. The meridian then flows upward at a slight angle to the shoulder crease then down to the forearm running along the inside edge of the large muscle, radial carpal flexor, of the foreleg, then under the carpus (wrist) and terminates at Lung 11 on the underside of the dewclaw.

Lung Meridian

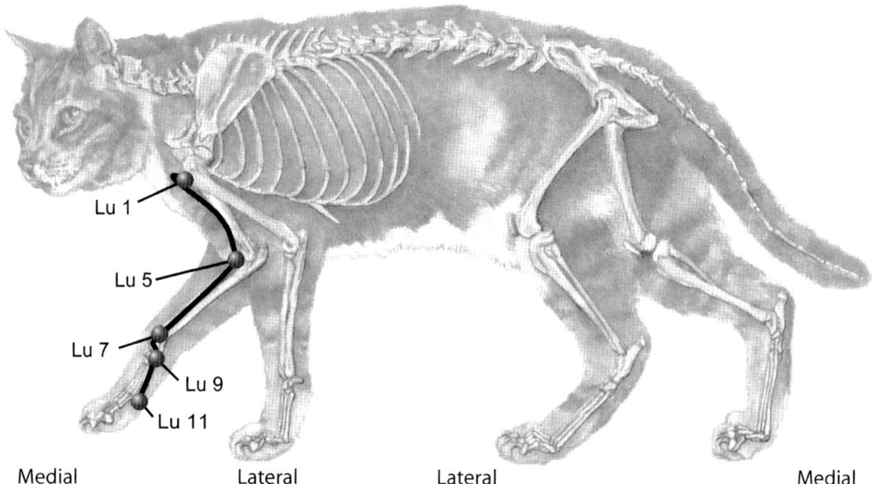

Point	Energetics/Function	Location
Lu 1	Alarm pt for Lu, regulates and tonifies Lung, clears Heat. Promotes descending of Lu chi. **Benefits** cough, asthma, immune regulation, shoulder or thoracic pain.	Located at the level of the 1st intercostal space, medial to the greater tubercle of the humerus, in the pectoral muscle.
Lu 5	Regulates and tonifies Lu, clears Heat, and redirects rebellious chi. **Benefits** high fever, vomiting, shoulder and elbow pain, diarrhea, dermatitis, immune-mediated skin disorders.	In cubital crease lateral to the tendon of biceps brachii muscle and medial to the tendon of the brachialis muscle.
Lu 7	Connecting pt. Regulates Lu, stimulates sweating, regulates CV. Master pt for head and neck. **Benefits** asthma, cough, facial paralysis, stiff neck, cervical spondylosis, and toothache.	Located proximal to the styloid process on the radius, 1.5 cun above the transverse crease of the carpus.
Lu 9	Source pt. Influential pt for arteries and pulse. Regulates and tonifies Lu, enriches Yin, clears Heat, redirects rebellious chi, & circulates Protective chi. **Benefits** chest pain, asthma, cough, shoulder and back pain, carpal joint pain, Lu deficiency, and heatstroke or coma.	Located on medial aspect of the radiocarpal joint, just cranial to the radial artery, at the level of Ht 7.
Lu 11	Jing-well pt. Revives consciousness, calms spirit, restores collapsed Yang. **Benefits** febrile conditions, cough, vomiting, fatigue, heatstroke, seizures, and disorientation.	Located on the medial side of the dewclaw (digit 1) of the front paw, at the nail bed.

Large Intestine
Foreleg *Yangming* / Yang Brightness
The Great Eliminator

The Large Intestine, in Chinese *Da Chang*, receives food and water from the Small Intestine. It is responsible for the temporary storage of material waste and absorption of some fluid before eliminating the stool. Cleansing the body of waste has both a physical and energetic dimension. The Large Intestine is an important part of moving stagnant chi down and out of the body. As the yang counterpart to the Lung, the Large Intestine meridian supports the respiratory and immune system functions of the Lung meridian.

Functions & Attributes

- Receives food and water from the Small Intestine
- Re-absorbs fluid, stores and excretes feces
- Descends chi
- Balances chi and blood
- Belongs to the Metal Element
- Optimal flow of Chi 5 – 7 AM

Health Issues

- Respiratory conditions
- Mobility of forelimb, neck, and head
- Lymphatic circulation
- Sensitivity to climate
- Dental problems
- Constipation or diarrhea
- Immune system weakness
- Allergies

Emotional Issues

- Chronic or long-term grief
- Compulsive behaviors
- Indifference or aloofness
- Stubbornness
- Restlessness

Location and Flow of the Large Intestine meridian

The Large Intestine meridian begins on the forelimb on the medial side of the second digit. It proceeds up the second metacarpal to the topside of the dewclaw and then up and across the carpus (wrist) to the craniolateral aspect of the radius bone to the transverse crease of the elbow. From the elbow it flows along the ventral aspect of the humerus to the point of the shoulder then up the ventral portion of the neck and on to the mandible (lower jaw). As it flows down toward the nose it crosses on to the maxilla (upper jaw) and ends at Large Intestine 20 at the lateral side of the base of the nose.

Large Intestine Meridian

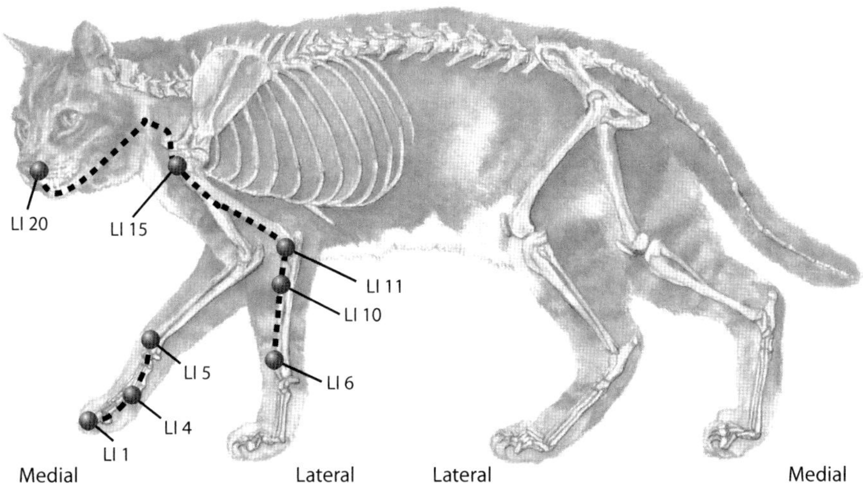

Point	Energetics/Function	Location
LI 1	Jing-well point. Clears Lung Heat, revives consciousness. **Benefits** nasal discharge, shoulder pain or lameness, and febrile issues.	On the medial side of the 2nd digit of the paw, at the nail bed.
LI 4	Source pt. Regulates and tonifies chi, alleviates pain, reduces fever, tonifies Protective chi. Master pt for face and mouth. **Benefits** neck, forelimb or shoulder pain, immunostimulation, immune mediated skin issues, expedites labor. Contraindicated in pregnancy.	Between the first (dewclaw) and 2nd metacarpal bones, on the medial side of the 2nd metacarpal.
LI 5	Dispels Wind Heat, clears Heat. **Benefits** skin disorders, carpal and dental pain. Calms the spirit.	In a depression on the craniomedial aspect of the radial carpal joint.

Large Intestine Meridian

Point	Energetics/Function	Location
LI 6	Clears Heat and dispels Wind. **Benefits** foreleg pain or stiffness, seizures, edema, and vision.	Craniolateral surface of the forelimb, in muscle groove between extensor carpi radialis and the common digital exensor muscles, 3 cun above LI 5.
LI 10	Regulates stomach and intestines, and reduces digestive stagnation. **Benefits** Chi deficiency, immuno-deficiency, diarrhea, abdominal pain, gingivitis, and generalized weakness.	On the craniolateral aspect of the thoracic limb, 2 cun below LI 11, in the groove between the extensor carpi radialis and the common digital extensor muscles.
LI 11	Tonification pt for deficiency patterns. Dispels Wind & Heat, builds Wei chi. **Benefits** elbow and forelimb issues, skin disorders, endocrine or febrile issues. Allergic or infectious diseases.	Lateral aspect of the thoracic limb, at the lateral end of the cubital crease. Find by flexing the elbow.
LI 15	Relaxes the sinews, dispels Wind and clears Heat. **Benefits** cervical pain, intervertebral issues, shoulder pain, and inflammation.	Found in front of and below the acromion on the front margin of the acromial head of the deltoid muscle.
LI 20	Dispels Wind. **Benefits** nasal obstruction, smell, paralysis, heat stoke, cough, sinusitis, fever, or cold.	At the widest part of the nostril, in the facial nasal labial groove.

Large Intestine Meridian

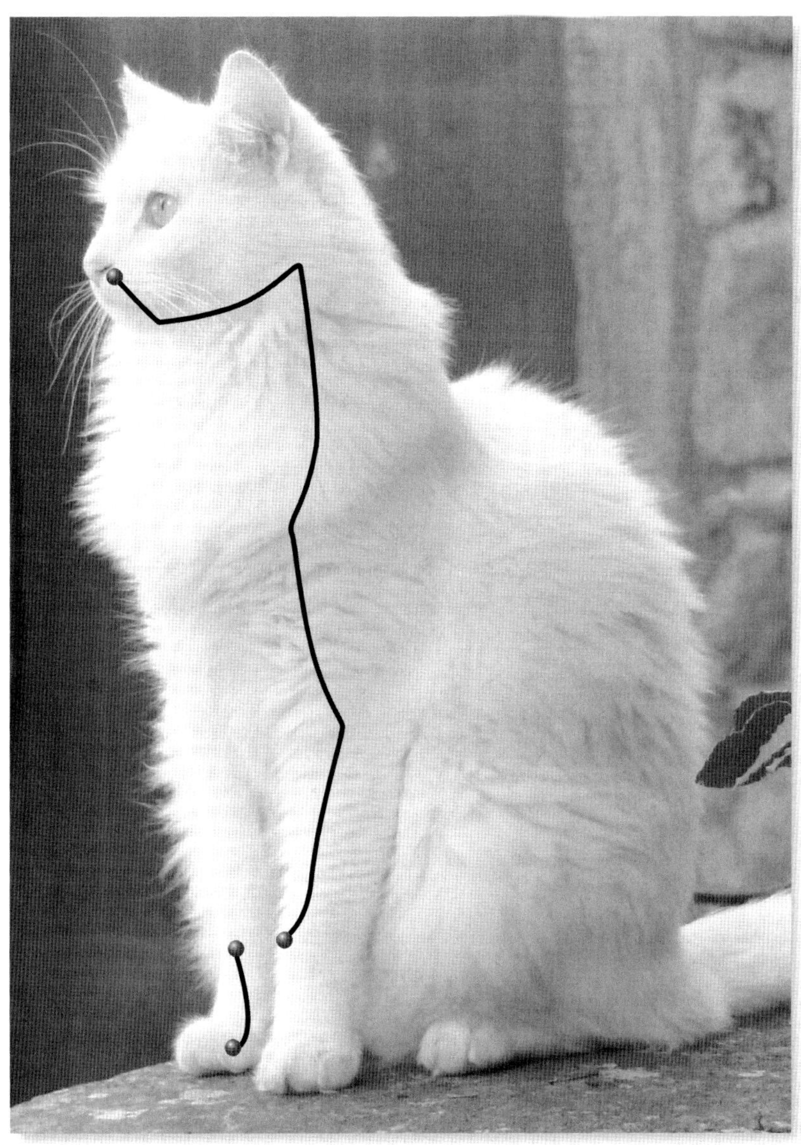

Stomach
Hind Leg *Yangming* / Yang Brightness
Sea of Nourishment

The Stomach, known in Chinese as *Wei*, is the origin of fluids and controls the digestion by "rotting and ripening" food. The Stomach and its paired yin organ system, the Spleen, act in concert to transform food into bio-absorbable nutrients and transport the nutrients to the Heart to be converted into blood and the Lung to be transformed into Protective chi (Wei chi). The nutrient-rich blood nourishes the muscles, the four limbs, and all of the body tissues. It is said that no matter what the disease if the Stomach chi is strong, the outlook is good; conversely, if the Stomach chi is low, the prognosis is not good.

Functions and Attributes

- Controls the "rotting and ripening" of food
- Controls the transportation of food
- Contributes to Protective chi
- Controls the descending of chi
- Originator of fluids
- Tonifies chi and blood
- Belongs to the Earth Element
- Optimal flow of Chi 7 – 9 AM

Health Issues

- Muscle tone or strength
- Digestive disorders
- Weight problems
- Stifle problems
- Abdominal distention or bloat
- Lethargy and low stamina
- TMJ tension and pain
- Unruly appetite
- Eye problems

Emotional Issues

- Anxiety, chronic nervous tension
- Excessive worry
- Lack of focus or awareness
- Overprotective behaviors
- Obsessive behaviors

Location and flow of the Stomach Meridian

Stomach 1 is located under the eye in the center of the lower lid. From this point, the meridian descends onto the muzzle then back to the corner of the cat's mouth. It swings up the jaw in front of the ear then dives down below the cervical vertebrae, through the front legs and travels along the nipple line to the end of the cat's ribs. At the end of the ribs the meridian moves closer to the ventral midline and continues to the hind leg. On the hind leg this meridian flows down the cranial edge on the lateral side of the leg past the hock to Stomach 45 on the lateral side of the third digit of the hind paw.

Stomach Meridian

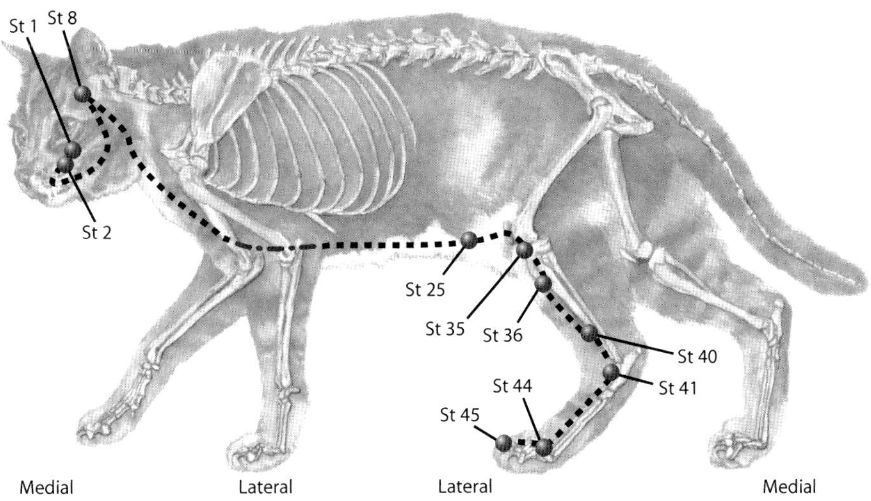

Point	Energetics/Function	Location
St 1	Brightens the eyes, dispels Wind, and clears Heat. **Benefits** conjunctivitis, uveitis, eye discharge, swelling, excessive tearing.	Directly below (ventral to) the center of the pupil.
St 2	Brightens the eyes, relaxes the sinews, dispels Wind and Cold. **Benefits** conjunctivitis, uveitis, and clears the nose.	Below St 1, in a depression at the center of the infraorbital foramen.
St 8	Dispels Wind, clears Heat, and brightens the eyes. **Benefits** eye discharge & blurred vision.	In a depression caudal to the supraorbital fossa, 1 cun toward the front edge of the ear base.
St 25	Alarm point of the large intestine. Regulates Spleen and Stomach, reduces digestive stagnation. **Benefits** gastrointestinal disorders, abdominal masses, diarrhea or constipation, vomiting, and IBD.	Found 2 cun lateral to the umbilicus.

Stomach Meridian

Point	Energetics/Function	Location
St 35	St 35 Dispels Wind, Cold, and clears Heat. **Benefits** stifle pain or inflammation, osteoarthritis, lower limb weakness.	In a depression distal to the patella and lateral to the patellar ligament.
St 36	Master point for GI and abdomen. Regulates, strengthens and tonifies the Spleen, regulates Stomach, tonifies nutritive chi, reduces digestive stagnation. Regulates and tonifies chi and blood. **Benefits** stomach pain, gastric ulcers, constipation, diarrhea, stifle pain, hind limb weakness, strengthens chi. Contraindicated in pregnancy.	Located 3 cun below St 35, one finger-breadth lateral to the tibial crest, in the lateral portion of the cranial tibial muscle.
St 40	Influential point for Phlegm. Connecting pt. Regulates Stomach and Intestines, and calms the spirit. **Benefits** depression, mania, anxiety, hind limb paralysis, and gastrointestinal disorders.	Found halfway between the lateral malleolus of the fibula and the top of the tibia, on the lateral aspect of the pelvic limb.
St 41	Regulates Stomach, dispels Wind, calms spirit, and clears the brain. **Benefits** seizures, depression, constipation, releases the hock, facial pain, pelvic limb issues.	On the cranial aspect of the hock in a depression on the midline, at the level of the lateral malleolus, between the tendons of long digital extensor and cranial tibialis muscles.
St 44	Regulates the St and Intestines, transforms Damp-Heat, regulates chi. **Benefits** febrile issues, poor appetite, gingivitis, hock pain, abdominal pain, or gastric ulcers.	On the hind limb, above the web margin, between the 3rd and 4th digits.
St 45	Jing-well point. Calms the spirit, regulates the St and clears Heat. **Benefits** seizures, abdominal pain, dental pain, and fever.	On the lateral side of the 3rd digit of the hind paw, at the nail bed.

Stomach Meridian

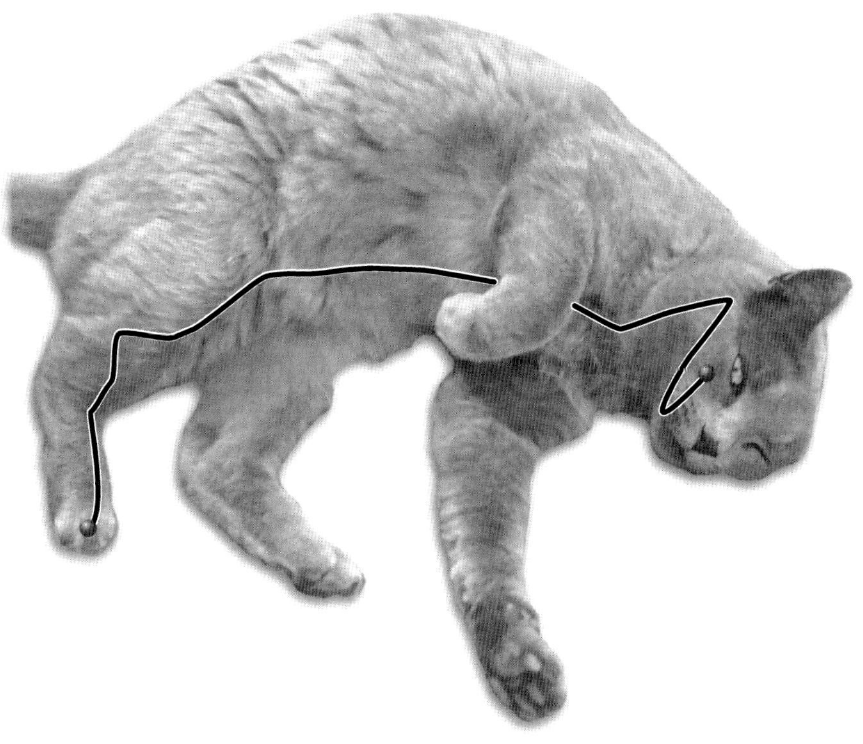

Spleen
Hind Leg *Taiyin* / Greater Yin
Controller of Distribution

The yin organ system, Spleen, along with the Stomach, are considered the "center within the body" and are essential to the creation of "Acquired chi." Acquired chi, also referred to as Post-Natal or Post-Heavenly chi, is necessary to sustain the cat's life after birth. The Spleen, called *Pi* in Chinese, transforms and transports refined food essence up to combine with *Zong*, or Chest chi and be converted into Nutrient / *Ying* chi, which is even further refined to become True chi. The pure, highly-refined "True chi" enriches blood. If the Spleen is not functioning properly the entire body can suffer from lack of nourishment leading to a chi and blood deficiency.

Functions and Attributes

- Governs transformation and transportation of food essence
- Controls the blood within the vessels
- Source of chi and blood
- Nourishes the muscles and four limbs
- Holds the internal organs in place
- Manifests in the lower muzzle
- Sensory orifice is the mouth
- Fluid is saliva
- Emotion is worry or over-thinking
- Belongs to the Earth Element
- Optimal flow of Chi 9 – 11 AM

Health Issues

- Muscle tone or strength
- Digestive disorders
- Weight problems
- Stifle problems
- Pain of the medial aspect of the stifle
- Abdominal distention / bloat
- Organ prolapse
- Edema / water retention
- Lethargy and low stamina
- Weak immune system
- TMJ tension and pain
- Unruly appetite

Emotional Issues

- Anxiety, excessive worry
- Lack of focus or awareness
- Overprotective behaviors
- Obsessive behaviors

Location and Flow of the Spleen Meridian

Spleen 1 is located on the medial side of the nail bed on the second digit of the hind paw. Most cats do not have a hind dewclaw which would be considered the first digit; if the cat has hind dewclaws, you may want to place Spleen 1 on the medial side of the nail bed of the dew claw. The Spleen meridian travels up the medial side of the hind leg going forward (cranial) passing in front of the medial malleolus of the tibia at the hock, then continuing up the leg on the caudal edge of the tibia to the stifle. It then flows cranially to the upper part of the hind leg to the inguinal groove and on to the ventral portion of the cat's abdomen. Once on the body it heads toward the front of the rib cage where it makes a sharp angle back toward the tail (caudal) to the sixth intercostal space, at about the level of the shoulder joint. This is where Spleen 21, the last point on the Spleen meridian is located.

Spleen Meridian

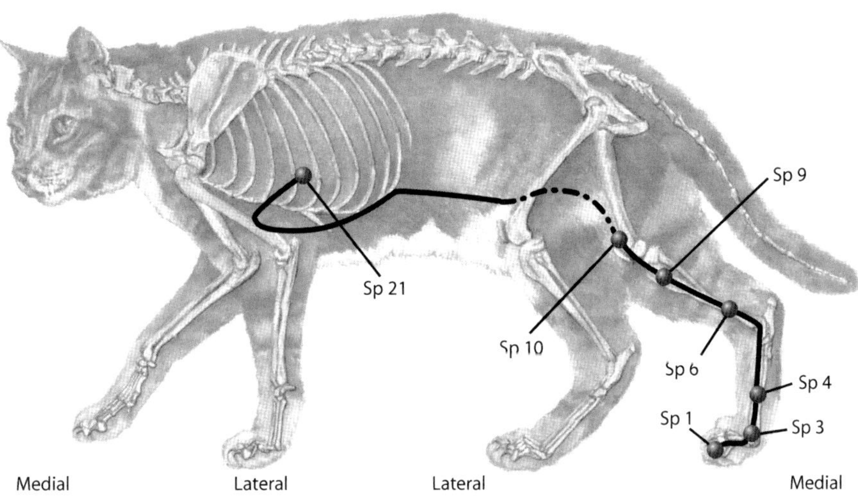

Point	Energetics/Function	Location
Sp 1	Jing-well point. Regulates and tonifies the Sp, facilitates blood flow, contains blood, calms spirit and clears brain. **Benefits** abdominal pain, distension, lack of appetite, convulsions and shock.	On the medial side of the 2nd digit of hind paw at the nail bed.
Sp 3	Source point. Regulates and strengthens Sp, regulates St and LI. **Benefits** diarrhea, constipation, digestion, and obesity.	Medial aspect of hind leg above the metatarsophalangeal joint on the medial side of 2nd metatarsal bone.
Sp 4	Connecting point. Regulates and strengthens Spleen, regulates St, invigorates blood. Calms spirit. **Benefits** indigestion, abdominal pain, diarrhea, and irregular cycles.	On the caudomedial aspect of hindleg, in depression below (distal to) base of the 2nd metatarsal bone.

Spleen Meridian

Point	Energetics/Function	Location
Sp 6	Master pt for urogenital system & caudal abdomen. Tonifies chi, blood, Kidneys, and Spleen. Regulates Liver and chi. **Benefits** hypothyroidism, edema, fatigued extremities, infertility, Yin deficiency, urinary incontinence, immune system. Contraindicated in pregnancy.	Found 3 cun above the tip of the medial malleolus on the caudal border of the tibia.
Sp 9	Regulates and strengthens Sp, regulates St and water pathways. **Benefits** Yin deficiency conditions, edema, urinary incontinence, stifle pain.	On the medial side of the pelvic limb in, a depression between the caudal border of the gastrocnemius muscle.
SP 10	Regulates and tonifies blood, facilitates blood flow. Sea of Blood pt. **Benefits** blood deficiency, blood Heat, blood stagnation, fever, irregular heat cycles.	With stifle flexxed, this point is found 2 cun above patella, medial aspect, in depression in front of the sartorius muscle.
Sp 21	Connecting pt for all Connecting Pts Pts. Regulates chi and blood, tonifies Nutritive Chi, controls all Yin meridians. **Benefits** generalized body pain, fatigue, lethargy and weakness, digestive disorders and back pain. Fills in gaps in chi.	On lateral aspect of chest, in the 6th intercostal space, at about the level of the point of the shoulder.

Their function is to have chi and blood flow … the harmonious flow of chi and blood in the channels brings nutrients to the body, balances yin and yang, invigorates tendons, bones, and joints.

— "Treatise on the Original Organs"
from *Miraculous Pivot*

Functions of the Meridian System

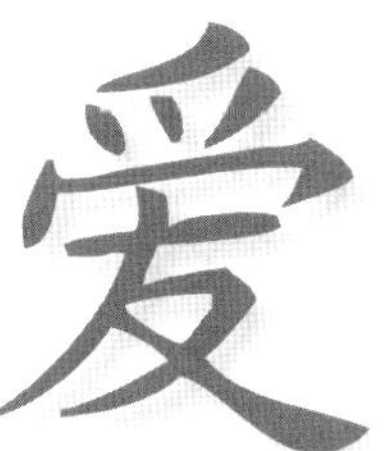

- The 12 Major Meridians are one continuous channel on which chi and blood (nourishing fluids) flow.
- Meridian energy shifts from yin to yang and yang to yin at the Jing-well points located on the nail beds and back pads of the cat's paws.
- Meridians are relatively superficial, they flow between skin and muscle tissue.
- Each individual meridian is connected to a specific internal organ and communicates the energy of that organ to the surface of the cat's body.
- When performing an acupressure session, you are accessing the energy of the internal organs by "working" with the meridians on the surface of the cat's body.

The Meridian System is responsible for:

1. Communication between the zang-fu organs
2. Connection of the entire of the body
3. Circulation of chi, blood, and other vital substances

Heart
Foreleg *Shaoyin* / Lesser Yin
Home of the Spirit

The Heart is known as the Monarch or Ruler of the entire body because of its important role in blood circulation. Heart chi must be vigorous to nourish the cat's body. Mental consciousness and the spirit of the animal (shen) is said to reside in the Heart as well. In Chinese thought, "consciousness" has a broader meaning and refers to the overall appearance and self-presentation of the cat. Consciousness has to do with the vitality of the animal.

When the cat is healthy and "strutting-his-stuff" we can tell. When a cat is sick, we know it immediately. The spirit, or shen, of the animal is said to be, "Housed in the Heart and Revealed in the eyes." Known in Chinese as *Xin*, the Heart is the yin organ system paired with the Small Intestine yang organ system.

Functions and Attributes

- Governs the direction and strength of blood flow and pulse
- Controls the blood vessels
- Regulates the nervous system
- Houses the mind and shen / spirit
- Regulates body heat
- Sensory orifice is the tongue
- Fluid is sweat or related to panting
- Emotion is joy
- Belongs to the Fire Element
- Optimal flow of Chi 11 AM – 1 PM

Health Issues

- Cardiovascular disorders
- Shoulder pain
- Atrophy, tension or swelling of the neck
- Brain or nervous system disorders
- Spontaneous or excessive panting
- Swollen or abnormal color of tongue

Emotional Issues

- Lack of joy / depression
- Lack of mental clarity or focus
- Mania / shen disturbance
- Restlessness and anxiety
- Nervous exhaustion

Location and Flow of the Heart Meridian:

Heart 1 is located under the foreleg on the cat's chest near the heart. From the chest this meridian flows on the inside (medial) and caudal edge of the foreleg and travels down the large muscle (digital flexor) until it turns into a tendon and begins to feel "ropey." Where the tendon begins the meridian flows to the lateral side of the leg and travels to the large space between the tendon attachment and the carpal bones of the wrist. The Heart meridian crosses the back of carpus (wrist), continues down the back edge of the fifth metacarpal to Heart 9 on the medial side of the fifth digit.

Heart Meridian

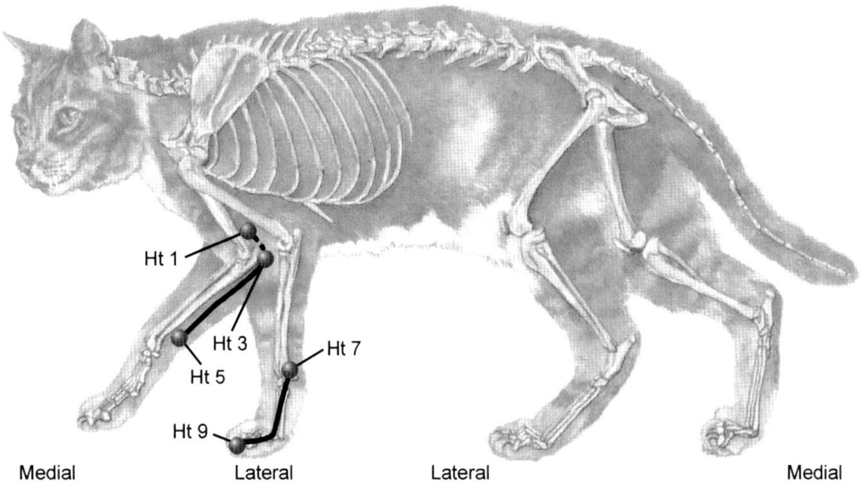

Point	Energetics/Function	Location
Ht 1	Regulates Ht, facilitates chi flow. **Benefits** shoulder lameness, Yin deficiency, and shen disturbances.	Center of axilla (armpit).
Ht 3	Regulates Ht, chi, and blood. Calms spirit and strengthens the brain. **Benefits** elbow, thoracic or Ht pain, seizures, and shen disturbances.	Medial side of elbow, between the end of the cubital crease and the medial epicondyle of the humerus.
Ht 5	Connecting pt. Regulates and tonifies Ht, and calms spirit. **Benefits** anxiety, fatigue, and carpal pain.	On the caudomedial aspect of the forelimb, about 1.5 cun above the carpus.
Ht 7	Source pt, cools Heat in blood, regulates and tonifies the Heart. **Benefits** anxiety, fever & chills, lack of appetite, epilepsy, behavioral issues.	At the transverse crease of the carpal joint, in a depression lateral to the flexor carpi ulnaris. Opposite Pe 7.
Ht 9	Jing-well pt. Revives consciousness and regulates the Heart. **Benefits** fever, shoulder & shen issues.	Medial side of the 5th digit of the front paw at the nail bed.

Small Intestine
Foreleg *Taiyang* / Greater Yang
Controller of Assimilation

The Small Intestine plays an important part in digestion. It receives the remains of the fluids and food not absorbed by the initial digestive process by the Stomach and Spleen. The Small Intestine is responsible for separating the clean from the turbid and absorbing the clean, usable fluids and nutrients. Hence, the Small Intestine, called *Xiao Chang* in Chinese, is instrumental in the assimilation of nutrients. This role of separating the pure from impure has further implications. The Small Intestine provides the capacity to discern right from wrong and the ability to distinguish relevant issues with clarity. The Small Intestine is the yang organ system paired with the Heart and in a way performs the role of keeping the monarch's kingdom of the body pure and offers clarity of mind to make fair, diplomatic judgments.

Functions & Attributes

- Controls receiving and transforming
- Separates clean from turbid
- Provides the power of discernment
- Regulates the function of the intestines
- Regulates the absorption of body fluids
- Belongs to the Fire Element
- Optimal flow of Chi 1 – 3 PM

Health Issues

- Arm, shoulder, and neck pain
- Atrophy, tension or swelling of the neck
- Digestion or absorption problems
- TMJ tension or pain
- Dental problems
- Urinary and bowel problems

Emotional Issues

- Not knowing right from wrong
- Lack of joy / depressed nature
- Lack of mental clarity or confusion
- Manic behavior / shen disturbance
- Restlessness and anxiety

Location and Flow of the Small Intestine Meridian

Small Intestine 1 is located at the nail bed on the lateral side of the fifth digit of the front paw. Staying on the caudolateral aspect of the metacarpals, this meridian travels up toward the body over the carpus, continues to the point of the elbow and on to the cat's body. Then it flows on to the scapula (shoulder blade) crossing to the neck and travels up the middle of the neck, over the mandible (lower jaw bone) to the to the maxilla (upper jaw bone) and then angles back to the soft spot at the base of the opening to the ear, Small Intestine 19.

Small Intestine Meridian

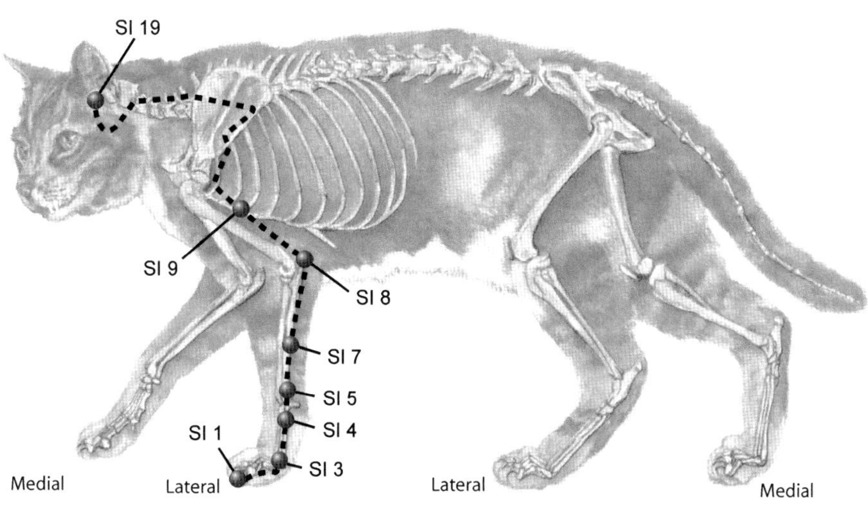

Point	Energetics/Function	Location
SI 1	Jing-well pt. Revives consciousness, opens sensory orifices. **Benefits** lactation, fever, coma, or shoulder pain.	On lateral aspect of the 5th digit of the front paw at the nail bed.
SI 3	Stimulates sweating, regulates GV, relaxes sinews, alleviates pain. **Benefits** joints, febrile issues, conjunctivitis, cervical and shoulder pain, epilepsy, and mania.	Just above the metacarpophalangeal joint of the 5th digit, on the lateral side.
SI 4	Source pt, relaxes sinews, clears Heat. **Benefits** carpal issues, cervical pain, and fever.	Lateral aspect of thoracic limb, below carpal joint, at base of 5th metacarpal bone.
SI 5	Clears Heat and dispels Wind Heat. Opens sensory orifices, calms the spirit, and clears the brain. **Benefits** convulsions, fright, tinnitus, fever, and carpal pain.	In a depression at the lateral styloid process of the radius, near the accessory carpal bone.
SI 7	Connecting pt, dispels Wind, calms the spirit, and clears the brain. **Benefits** pain in elbow and foreleg, cervical pain, or anxiety.	On the lateral aspect of the forelimb about 5/12ths the distance from the carpus to the cubital fossa.

Small Intestine Meridian

Point	Energetics/Function	Location
SI 8	Dispels Wind and relaxes the sinews. **Benefits** elbow pain, seizures, neck, shoulder and dental pain.	Medial side of the elbow between the humeral epicondyle and the olecranon.
SI 9	Dispels Wind. **Benefits** pain, stiffness, paralysis, arthritis of scapula, shoulder,	Caudal to the humerus in a large depression along the caudal border of deltoid muscle, at the level of the neck, and forearm. Reduces shoulder joint.inflammation.
SI 19	Clears Heat, opens the ears, and calms the spirit. **Benefits** auditory dysfunction, otitis, seizures, mania, or anxiety. of the ear.	Found in the depression rostral (toward front of head) to the tragus (projection at base of external ear)

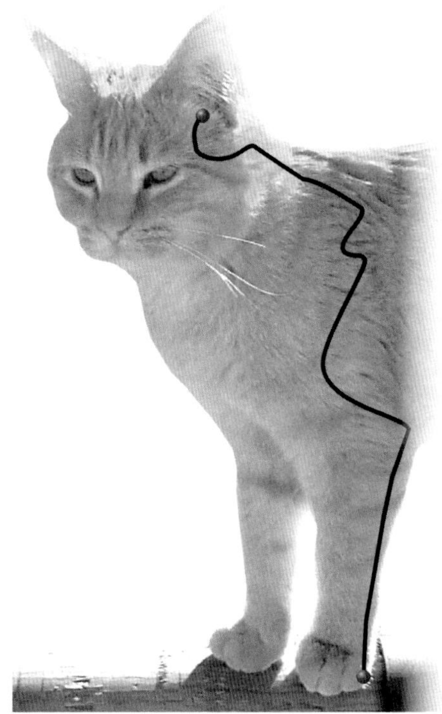

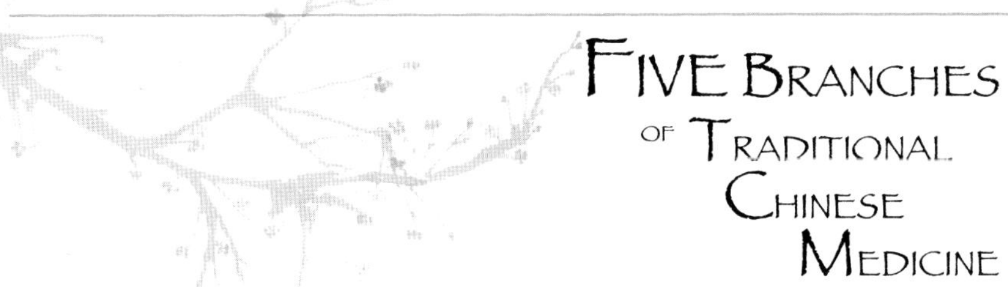

Five Branches of Traditional Chinese Medicine

From the perspective of this ancient medicine, everything is "medicine." Health is defined as both an internal and external balance of nutrients and energy so that the human and cat alike can function optimally within its environment. The intention is to support the body's capacity to adapt to constant change.

To achieve health and wellbeing, Chinese medicine incorporates five branches, or stems, as a guide to living a balanced life. Diet is essential. Exercise and body movement to enliven energy is absolutely necessary. All mammals need touch for sensory and caring stimulation. When imbalance threatens, further medicinal herbs and acupuncture and/or acupressure are necessary to restore the harmonious flow of chi and blood.

Five Branches of Traditional Chinese Medicine needed for a long, healthy life are:

- Diet
- Chi Gong – Exercise
- Tui Na – Chinese Meridian Acupressure-Massage
- Acupuncture
- Herbs

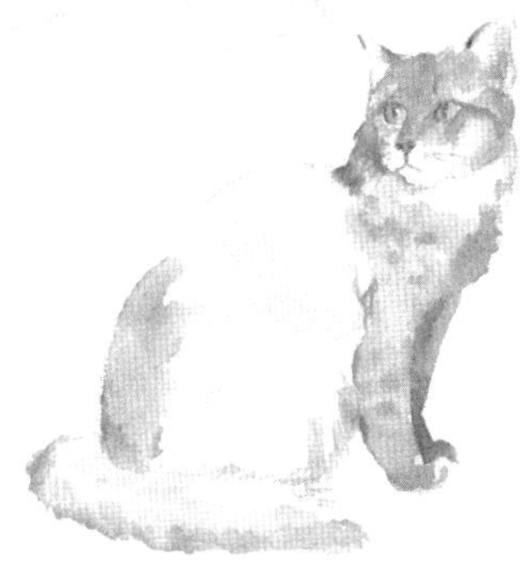

Bladder
Hind Leg *Taiyang* / Greater Yang
Great Mediator

The Bladder is responsible for body fluids, keeping the Lung moist, plus storage and excretion of urine. This yang organ system is paired with the Kidney and dominated by the Kidney. In Chinese the Bladder is known as *Pang Guang.*

Unlike the other 12 Major Meridians, the Bladder Meridian has two superficial branches with acupoints that flow on the dorsal aspect of the cat's back. The most medial branch, or channel, has a unique classification of acupoints called the Association points, or Back Shu points, since these 12 acupoints are directly related to the organ system for which each is named. For instance, Bladder 13 is the Lung Association point and Bladder 15 is the Heart Association point. Because these acupoints are connected to an organ system, we can use these points for both assessment and point work during the acupressure routine.

Functions and Attributes

- Stores fluids and excretes urine
- Removes fluid by chi transformation
- Belongs to the Water Element
- Optimal flow of Chi 3 – 5 PM

Health Issues

- Urinary tract problems
- Back and lower back Soreness
- Dry lungs
- Low physical energy
- Body fluid problems

Emotional Issues

- Excessive or chronic anxiety
- Fear issues
- Jealousy

Location and Flow of the Bladder Meridian

Bladder 1 is located at the inner canthus (corner) of the eye. From there, the Bladder meridian runs up and over the top of the cat's head, down the neck, and over the withers close to the midline. On the caudal side of the scapula, the meridian divides into two channels. The inner branch is 1.5 cun lateral and the outer branch is 3 cun lateral to the dorsal midline. Both branches flow down the back toward the tail. The inner branch continues down the caudal edge of the hind leg traveling in and along the crease of the biceps femoris and semitendinosus muscles down to Bladder 67 on the lateral side of the fifth digit. The Bladder meridian is one of the longest meridians on the body running from head to hind paw.

Bladder Meridian

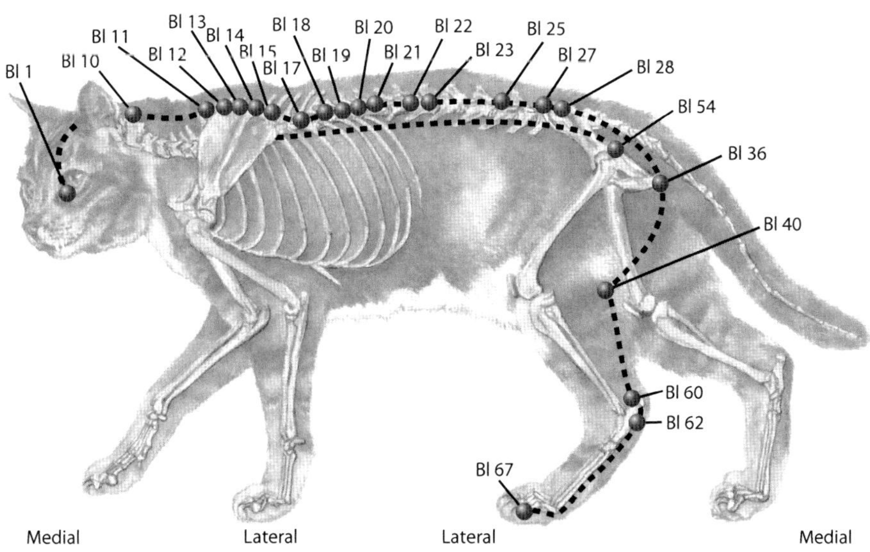

Point	Function/Energetics	Location
Bl 1	Opens and brightens the eyes, dispels Wind, clears Fire & Heat. Enriches Yin. **Benefits** all eye disorders including uveitis, conjunctivitis, myopia, and optic nerve atrophy.	In the indentation dorsal to the medial canthus of the eye.
Bl 10	Opens sensory orifices, dispels Wind, and Cold, clears Heat. **Benefits** the eyes, nasal congestion, back pain, neck injuries, epilepsy, and intervertebral disc disease.	1.5 cun off the dorsal midline, in a depression caudal to the wing of the atlas.
Bl 11	Influential pt for bone. Relaxes sinews, strengthens bone and joints. **Benefits** osteoarthritis, intervertebral disc disease, cervical pain, thoracic limb lameness, and most joint issues.	1.5 cun lateral to the dorsal midline, at the cranial edge of the scapula.

Bladder Meridian

Point	Energetics/Function	Location
Bl 12	Influential pt wind and trachea. Regulates the Lu, dispels Wind. **Benefits** cervical and thoracic pain, nasal congestion, or fever.	1.5 cun lateral to caudal border of dorsal spinous process of the 2nd thoracic vertebra.
Bl 13	Association pt for Lu. Regulates and tonifes the Lung. **Benefits** any respiratory condition, Yin deficiency, neck or back stiffness.	1.5 cun lateral to the caudal border of the dorsal spinous process of the 3rd thoracic vertebra.
Bl 14	Association pt for Pe. Regulates and tonifies the Ht, helps spread Liver chi. **Benefits** anxiety, palpitations, cough, or heart irregularities.	1.5 cun lateral to the caudal border of the dorsal spinous process of 4th thoracic vertebra.
Bl 15	Association pt for Ht. Regulates and tonifies the Ht, cools Heat in blood, calms the spirit, strengthens and clears brain. **Benefits** cardiac disorders, pain or palpitations, seizures or disorientation.	1.5 cun lateral to the caudal border of the dorsal spinous process of the 5th thoracic vertebra.
Bl 17	Influential pt for blood and diaphragm. Regulates and tonifies Sp and blood, and enriches Yin. **Benefits** the diaphragm, nonresponsive skin disorders, fever, low hemoglobin, white blood count, or any condition of the blood.	1.5 cun lateral to the caudal border of the dorsal spinous process of the 7th thoracic vertebra.
Bl 18	Association pt for Liver. Regulates and tonifies Liver, regulates GB, facilitates chi flow, and brightens the eyes. **Benefits** Liver, GB, or any eye condition, seizures, chronic fatigue, and Liver chi stagnation.	1.5 cun lateral to the caudal border of the dorsal spinous process of the 10th thoracic vertebra.
Bl 19	Association pt for GB. Regulates Liv and GB, clears Heat. **Benefits** Liv Yang rising, Liv chi stagnation,low fever, any eye disorder, sciatica, intervertebral disc issues. Expels parasites.	1.5 cun lateral to the caudal border of the dorsal spinous process of the 11th thoracic vertebra.

Bladder Meridian

Point	Energetics/Function	Location
Bl 20	Association pt for Sp. Regulates & tonifies Spleen, tonifies Nutritive Chi and blood, reduces digestive stagnation. **Benefits** edema, diarrhea, anemia, gastrointestinal disorders, pain of the medial stifle, insufficient lactation, hard abdominal masses.	1.5 cun lateral to the caudal border of the dorsal spinous process of 12th thoracic vertebra.
Bl 21	Association pt for St. Regulates Stomach and tonifies the Spleen. **Benefits** gastrointestinal issues, edema, acute and chronic diarrhea, mid-back, stifle, and hind limb pain, or general weakness. Relieves vomiting.	1.5 cun lateral to the caudal border of the dorsal spinous process of the 13th thoracic vertebra.
Bl 22	Association pt for TH. Regulates TH and tonifies Ki, resolves dampness. **Benefits** chronic nephritis, urinary issues, hormonal imbalances, edema, and disc issues.	1.5 cun lateral to the caudal border of the dorsal spinous process of the 1st lumbar vertebra.
Bl 23	Association pt for Ki. Tonifies Ki Essence, warms Yang, and tonifies Source Chi. **Benefits** general weakness, seizures, ears and eyes, lower back pain, concentration, renal issues, the brain, estrous cycles, and impotence.	1.5 cun lateral to the caudal border of the dorsal spinous process of the 2nd lumbar vertebra.
Bl 25	Association pt for LI. Regulates LI, warms Cold. **Benefits** diarrhea or constipation, lumbar pain and disc issues, and abdominal pain, and all intestinal disorders.	1.5 cun lateral to the caudal border of the dorsal spinous process of the 5th lumbar vertebra.
Bl 26	Gate of Source Chi. Strengthens Ki Yang and Chi. **Benefits** urinary incontinence, lower back pain, sciatica, constipation or diarrhea, impotence.	1.5 cun lateral to the caudal border of the dorsal spinous process of 6th lumbar vertebra.

Bladder Meridian

Point	Energetics/Function	Location
Bl 27	Association pt for SI. Regulates SI, stabilizes Essence. **Benefits** lower back and abdominal pain, and urinary issues.	1.5 cun lateral to the caudal border of the dorsal spinous process of the 7th lumbar vertebra.
Bl 28	Association pt for Bl. Regulates Bl, and water pathways, clears Heat. **Benefits** urinary issues, constipation and diarrhea, and cauda equina.	Located lateral to the 2nd foramen, in a depression between the sacrum and the medial border of the dorsal iliac spine.
Bl 35	Clears Heat. **Benefits** tail paralysis, pain, and bloody diarrhea.	In crease lateral to the tail base, 1.5 cun off the sacrocaudal dorsal midline.
Bl 36	Strengthens lower back and moves chi. **Benefits** lumbosacral pain, paralysis, and perianal disorders.	Below the ischial tuberosity, at the pelvic limb proximal end of the muscle groove between the biceps femoris and the semitendinosus muscles.
Bl 39	Regulates TH, Bl, and water pathways. **Benefits** urinary incontinence, edema, hock pain, nephritis, or lower back pain.	Lateral end of popliteal crease, just above and cranial to Bl 40.
Bl 40	Master point for back and hips. Dispels Wind, clears Heat, alleviates pain, and revives consciousness. **Benefits** low back and hips, strengthens stifles, urinary incontinence, autoimmune disease, spondylosis, hip joint pain, caudal paresis or paralysis.	Located at the midpoint of the transverse crease of the popliteal fossa.
Bl 54	Strengthens lower back and resolves Damp Heat. **Benefits** hip joint pain, pelvic limb lameness and muscle atrophy, and sciatica.	Just above (dorsal to) the greater trochanter of the femur.

Bladder Meridian

Point	Energetics/Function	Location
Bl 60	Facilitates chi and blood flow, regulates invigorates blood, dispels Wind Cold. **Benefits** seizures, lower back and sacral pain and stiffness, hock pain, hypertension. Expedites labor. Contraindicated in pregnancy.	Caudolateral aspect of the hind limb, at the thin fleshy tissue at the hock, opposite Ki 3.
Bl 62	Clears Fire and Heat, dispels Wind and Cold, calms the spirit. **Benefits** ataxia, weakness of all four limbs, ocular disorders, fatigue, and disorientation.	Lateral side of the hock, in a depression directly below the lateral malleolus.
Bl 67	Jing-well point. Regulates chi and blood, dispels Wind, clears Heat. Clears nose and brightens the eyes. **Benefits** ocular issues, nasal disorders, expedites labor, calms and repositions fetus. Contraindicated in pregnancy.	Lateral aspect of the 5th digit of the hind paw, at the nail bed.

Bladder Meridian

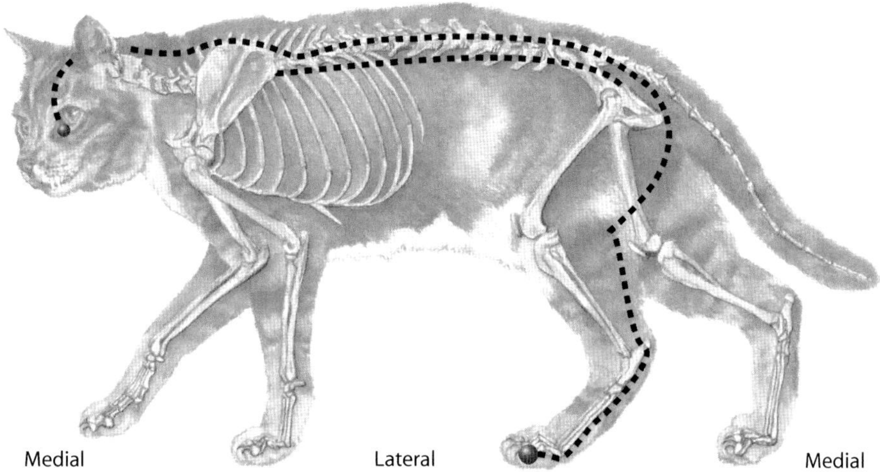

Kidney
Hind Leg *Shaoyin* / Lesser Yin
Residence of Resolution

The Kidney organ system is called the "Root of Life" because it stores the substantive foundation of the cat's life. The Kidney stores Original, or Source, Chi. Kidney chi is the original yin and yang of the body that the kitten inherits from the queen and the tom. It is the Jing, or essence, with which the kitten arrives on earth and depletes over the years until it can go no further and death ensues. Essence Chi determines the physical and emotional strength and constitutional vitality of the cat.

The relationship of the Kidney and the Lung is significant and forms the inner core strength of the body. Lung chi descends and Kidney chi must be strong enough to grasp and "root the breath." The animal's will power, *zhi*, reflects this core strength in his force of determination.

Kidney, *Shen* in Chinese, is the yin organ system paired with the Bladder which is yang. Together they are heavily involved in the functioning of the body's water metabolism.

Functions and Attributes:

- Stores *Jing Chi* / Essence chi
- Governs birth, growth, reproduction and development
- Produces marrow and fills the brain
- Controls bones and manufactures blood
- Dominates water metabolism
- Controls the reception and grasping of Lung chi
- Controls the lower two orifices
- Houses will power
- Manifests in the quality of fur
- Sensory orifice is the ear
- Fluid is heavy phlegm (spittle)
- Emotion is fear
- Belongs to the Water Element
- Optimal flow of Chi 5 – 7 PM

Health Issues

- Lower back and back pain
- Hock and stifle problems
- Bone and arthritis issues
- Lack of physical energy
- Urinary tract problems
- Reproductive and estrous cycle problems
- Development issues
- Dental issues
- Loss of hearing
- Ear problems

Emotional Issues

- Excessive or chronic anxiety
- Fear issues
- Jealousy

Location and Flow of the Kidney Meridian

Kidney 1 is located on the hind paw behind the central, large pad. The meridian runs up the caudomedial aspect of the leg to the hock. It then circles the hock and continues to flow up the medial aspect of the leg to the inguinal groove, or groin area, then on to the ventral abdomen about 1 cun parallel to the midline along the chest. The last acupoint on the Kidney meridian is Kidney 27, which is located between the breastbone (sternum) and first rib.

Kidney Meridian

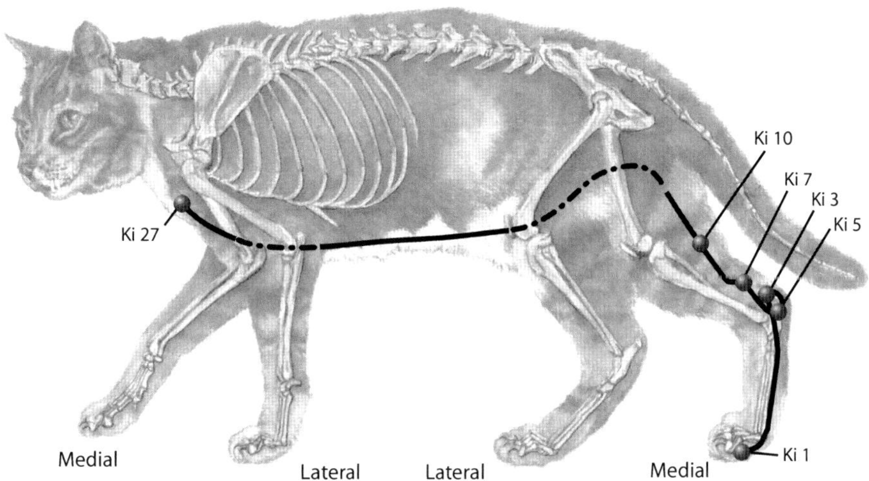

Point	Energetics/Function	Location
Ki 1	Jing-well point. Restores Yang, revives consciousness. **Benefits** infertility, urinary incontinence, seizures, heatstroke, and fever.	On the plantar surface of hind paw, at the back (caudal) edge of the metatarsal footpad.
Ki 3	Source pt. Tonifies Ki, Source chi, blood and Essence, restores collapsed Yin, calms fetus, and strengthens the brain. **Benefits** arthritis, local swelling of hock, lower back pain, kidney dysfunction, ears, irregular estrous cycles, chronic renal failure.	In a depression between the medial malleolus of the tibia and the calcaneal tendon. Opposite Bl 60.
Ki 5	Tonifies the Kidneys and regulates the bladder. **Benefits** irregular estrous, anestrous, and frequent urination.	One cun distal (below) Ki 3, caudal to the distal end of the tibia on the caudomedial side of the pelvic limb.

Kidney Meridian

Point	Energetics/Function	Location
Ki 7	Tonifies Ki, and Protective Chi, enriches Yin, regulates water pathways, unblocks pulses. **Benefits** lower back and Ki pain, edema, diarrhea, pelvic limb paresis or paralysis.	Caudomedial aspect of the pelvic limb, 2 cun proximal to Ki 3, on the cranial border of the Achilles tendon.
Ki 10	Tonifies Ki, clears Heat and Heat in blood. **Benefits** impotence, stifle pain, or lower abdominal pain.	Medial side of the popliteal fossa at the level of Bl 40, between the semimembranosus and the semitendinosus muscles.
Ki 27	Association pt of all Association pts. Tonifies Ancestral Chi and Ki, regulates Lu and St, redirects rebellious chi downward, warms Cold. **Benefits** immune-mediated issues, cough, disorientation, anxiety, vomiting, lack of appetite, or thoracic pain.	Found between the sternum and the 1st rib, 2 cun lateral to the ventral midline.

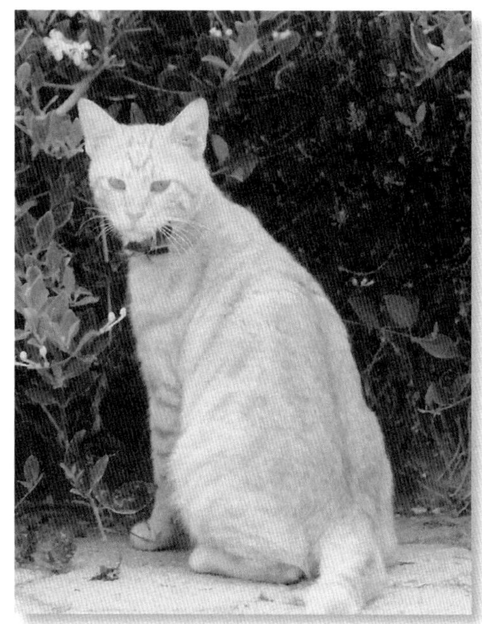

Pericardium
Foreleg *Jueyin* / Absolute Yin
Heart Protector

The Pericardium, *Xin Bao* in Chinese, is the sheathing surrounding the heart. Since the Heart is the Monarch of the body, the Pericardium's role is to protect the Heart from physical and emotional insult. As the Heart Protector, the Pericardium is an active agent of the Heart in assisting the Heart in all of its functions and is often used as a surrogate for the Heart.

Many of the Chinese texts do not consider the Pericardium an organ system but rather an appendage to the Heart. However, the yin Pericardium meridian and its associated acupoints are as powerful and commonly used as any of the 12 Major Meridians and their acupoints. The Pericardium is paired with the yang Triple Heater organ system.

Functions and Attributes

- Protects the Heart from external or internal pathogens
- Assists the Heart in cardiovascular functions
- Assists in balancing emotions
- Emotion is trust / intimacy
- Belongs to the Fire Element
- Optimal flow of Chi 7 – 9 PM

Health Issues

- Chest pain or tension
- Forelimb pain or soreness
- Cardiovascular problems
- Blood stasis or deficiency

Emotional Issues

- Bonding difficulty
- Lack of trust
- Mental clarity
- Timidity
- Abandonment issues
- Anxiety

Location and Flow of the Pericardium Meridian

The Pericardium meridian begins deep within the body at the sac that surrounds the heart. Pericardium 1 is located where the meridian surfaces near the fifth rib at the medial aspect of the elbow and just lateral to the nipple line. It then travels down the middle of the medial aspect of the foreleg to the accessory carpal bone. The meridian continues down the back inside of the lower leg, along the flexor tendon, to Pericardium 9, the last point on this meridian.

Pericardium Meridian

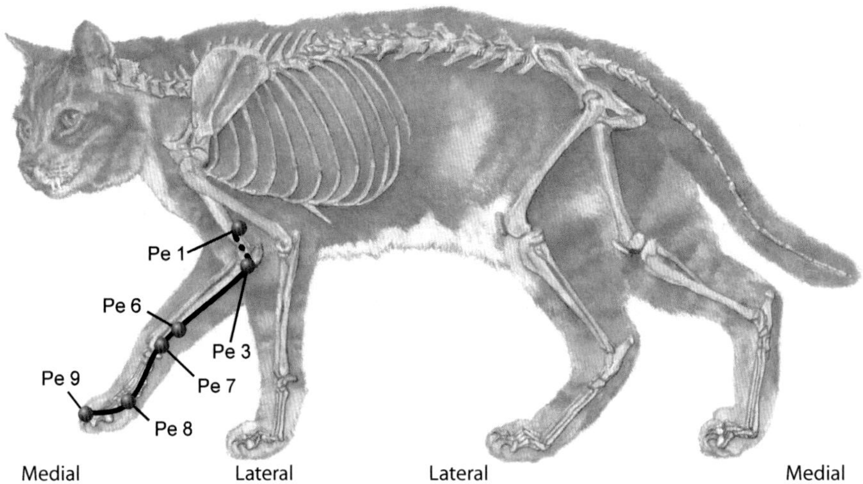

Point	Energetics/Function	Location
Pe 1	Regulates chi, clears Heat, expands the chest. **Benefits** cough, fatigued extremities, insufficient lactation or mastitis.	In the 5th intercostal space, medial to the point of the elbow.
Pe 3	Regulates Heart, St, and intestines. Clears Heat. **Benefits** heatstroke, febrile diseases, cardiac arrhythmias, shoulder and elbow pain, and diarrhea.	Medial side of the cubital crease of the elbow, just in back of the tendon of the biceps brachii muscle.
Pe 6	Connecting pt, Master pt for chest and cranial abdomen. Regulates and tonifies Ht, facilitates chi flow, calms the spirit and clears brain, spreads Liv chi, invigorates blood, sends rebellious chi downward. **Benefits** seizures, shen disturbances, severe agitation, nausea, vomiting, and palpitations.	2 cun above the transverse crease of the carpus, between the tendons of the superficial digital flexor and the flexor carpi radialis. Opposite TH 5.

Pericardium Meridian

Point	Energetics/Function	Location
Pe 7	Source pt. Regulates Heart and St, calms spirit and brain, cools Heat in blood. **Benefits** epilepsy, febrile issues, relieves anxiety, or vomiting. Local point for carpal pain.	Caudal to the tendon of the flexor carpi radialis and directly above the carpal bone.
Pe 8	Regulates Heart, cools Heat in blood, revives consciousness, and clears the brain. **Benefits** febrile diseases, gingivitis, shen disturbances, and anxiety.	Palmar side of the thoracic limb, under the large center pad, between the 3rd and 4th metacarpal bones.
Pe 9	Jing-well pt. Regulates Ht, revives consciousness, restores collapsed Yang. **Benefits** febrile diseases, heatstroke, shock, and lack of consciousness.	Lateral side of the 3rd digit of the front paw, at the nail bed.

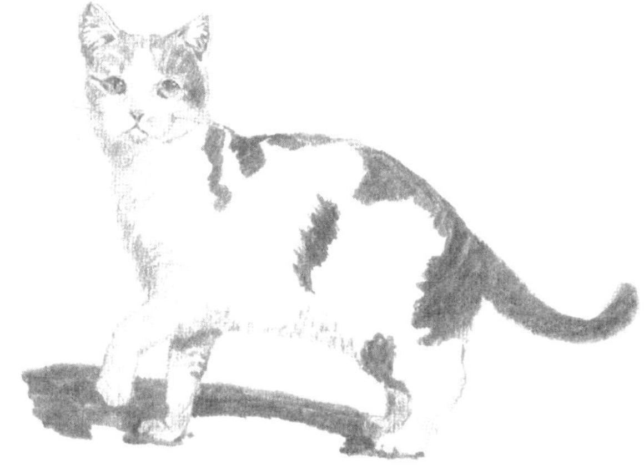

Triple Heater
Foreleg *Shaoyang* / Lesser Yang
Commander of All Energies

The Triple Heater, known in Chinese as *San Jiao*, is an esoteric aspect of Chinese medicine. It is viewed as an energetic organ and a functional system. As an energetic organ it does not have a tangible form. The Triple Heater is responsible for transforming and transporting chi so that it flows unimpeded to all parts of the body. In this role, it assists in transforming and transporting nourishment and excreting waste as well as directing chi to all the organs. As an organ, it is the largest of the body dividing the trunk into three distinct compartments. The upper "burner" includes the Lung, Heart and Pericardium. The middle burner includes the Spleen and Stomach. And, the lower burner includes the Large and Small Intestine, Gall Bladder, Liver, Kidney and Bladder. The Triple Heater is responsible for all of the organs working in concert with each other.

The Triple Heater is called "the Avenue of Original Chi" because of its role in transporting Original Chi to the 12 Major Meridians. The Original Chi resides in the Kidney and is transported by the Triple Heater where it surfaces at the Source points on each meridian. The Triple Heater is also involved in the functioning of the body's lymphatic system. It is a complex organ system and warrants much study. The Pericardium is the yin meridian paired with the Triple Heater.

Functions and Attributes

- Directs Original chi to the organs and Source points
- Coordinates the three energetic compartments
- Responsible for "thermo-regulation"
- Regulates water passages
- Belongs to the Fire Element
- Optimal flow of Chi 9 – 11 PM

Health Issues

- Forelimb, neck, and head pain or soreness
- Immune system issues (lymphatic system)
- Temporomandibular (TMJ) problems
- Ear problems / deafness
- Eye issues
- Temperature regulation
- Climate sensitivity
- Stiff neck and head
- Metabolic problems
- Edema

Emotional Issues

- Depression
- Nervous anxiety

Location and flow of the Triple Heater Meridian

Triple Heater 1 is located on the foreleg at the lateral side of the nail bed of the fourth digit of the cat's paw. The meridian flows up the metacarpals on the lateral aspect of the foreleg, to the carpus (wrist) and continues up the middle of the radius bone to the elbow. It continues along the lateral side of the thoracic limb to the shoulder area. From here it courses up the scapula and continues along the lateral aspect of the neck below the vertebrae to the base of the ear. Then it flows up behind the ear and down to the top of the jaw and over to the depression slightly above the lateral border of the eye to Triple Heater 23, the last point on this meridian.

Triple Heater Meridian

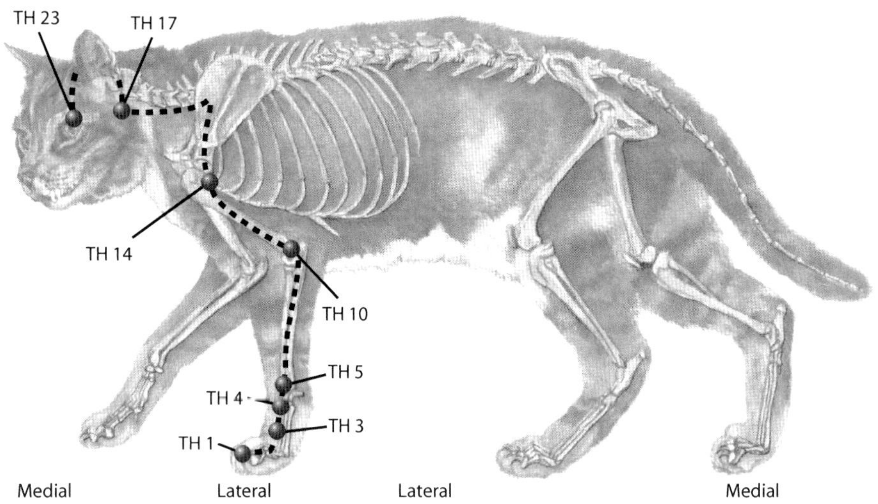

Point	Energetics/Function	Location
TH 1	Jing-well pt. Dispels Wind, revives consciousness, opens sensory orifices. **Benefits** fever, conjunctivitis, deafness, tinnitus, or shoulder pain.	Lateral side of the 4th digit of the front paw, at the nail bed.
TH 3	Clears Heat, dispels Wind. **Benefits** ear and eye disorders, fever, shoulder pain, local joint pain.	On the dorsum of the foot, on the lateral side of the 4th metacarpal bone, near the metacarpophalangeal joint.
TH 4	Source pt. Dispels Wind, clears Fire. **Benefits** swelling and pain of carpus, cold, fatigue, relieves shoulder and forelimb pain.	Lateral side of the forelimb, at the radiocarpal joint, cranial to the tendon of the common digital extensor.
TH 5	Connecting pt. Regulates TH, clears Heat, tonifies Protective chi, and alleviates pain. **Benefits** fevers, conjunctivitis, otitis, carpal, shoulder and cervical pain, and thoracic limb lameness.	Located 2 cun above the carpus, at the distal end of the interosseous space between the radius and the ulna.

Triple Heater Meridian

Point	Energetics/Function	Location
TH 10	Dispels Wind, clears Heat, calms spirit, and clears brain. **Benefits** cervical and dental pain, limb paresis or paralysis, or ear issues.	In a depression on the triceps tendon, just above the olecranon.
TH 14	Dispels Wind and Cold. **Benefits** all shoulder conditions, thoracic limb pain and lameness.	Behind the acromion of the scapula, on the deltoid muscle.
TH 17	Clears sensory orifices, dispels Wind relaxes facial sinews. **Benefits** all ear disorders, convulsions, TMJ, cervical pain, facial paralysis and swelling.	In a depression behind the base of the ear, between the mandible and the mastoid process.
TH 23	Brightens eyes, clears Heat, dispels Wind. **Benefits** all eye disorders, facial paralysis, dental diseases, or epilepsy.	In a depression at the end of the eyebrow on the rim of the eye orbit.

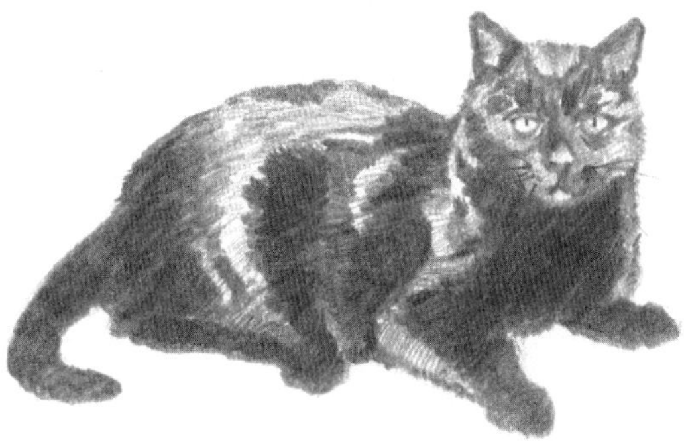

Triple Heater Meridian

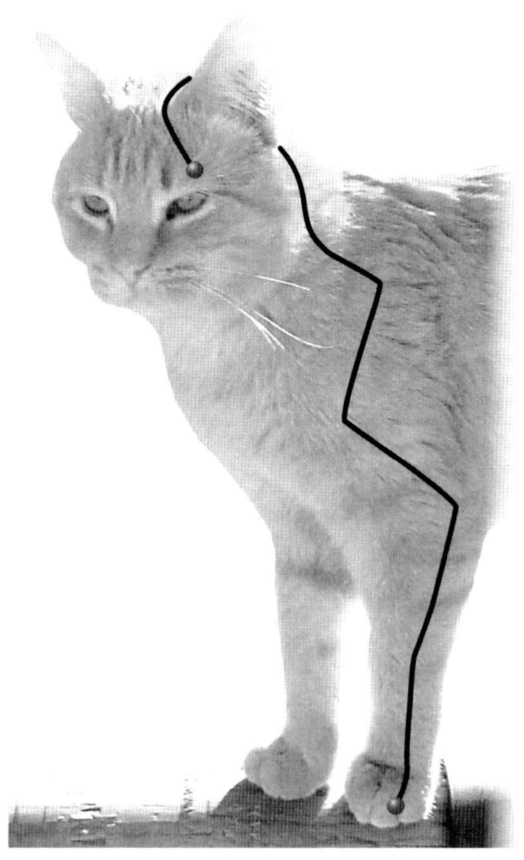

Gall Bladder
Hind Leg *Shaoyang* / Lesser Yang
Official of Decision-making and Judgment

The Gall Bladder stores and excretes bile as needed for digestion. This yang organ system is paired with the Liver, a yin organ system. The functions of the Gall Bladder are closely related to the Liver's capacity to provide a harmonious flow of chi. Known in Chinese as *Dan*, the Gall Bladder assists the Liver in many of its functions. This organ system is thought to affect the animal's courage and ability to take initiative and make decisions. Many physical issues can be addressed using the Gall Bladder meridian because it is one of the longest meridians in the body, extending from the head to the hind paw.

Functions and Attributes

- Stores and excretes bile
- Governs decision-making / judgment
- Assists in Liver functions
- Belongs to the Wood Element
- Optimal flow of Chi 11PM – 1AM

Health Issues

- Digestive disorders
- Muscle spasms, seizures, convulsions
- Tendon related pain or disorders
- Nail or claw problems
- Stiff or cramped muscles
- Vision or eye issues
- Neck, shoulder, hip, stifle, and hock problems
- Toxic issues

Emotional Issues

- Depression
- Lack of initiative
- Indecisiveness
- Aggressiveness or anger

Location and Flow of the Gall Bladder Meridian

Gall Bladder 1 is located at the outer canthus (corner) of the eye and flows upward to the medial side of the ear and over the head toward the occipital crest, then back over the head to the indent above the middle of the cat's eye. From there the meridian flows caudally over the cats head and down the dorsal aspect of the neck to the middle of the scapula. It passes under the scapula to the chest and travels over the abdomen. Then the meridian runs to the pelvic area, below the point of the hip to the hip joint. From the hip joint, the meridian traces down the midline of the lateral aspect of the thigh, down the femur, tibia, and metatarsals to the lateral side of the fourth digit of the hind paw terminating on Gall Bladder 44.

Gall Bladder Meridian

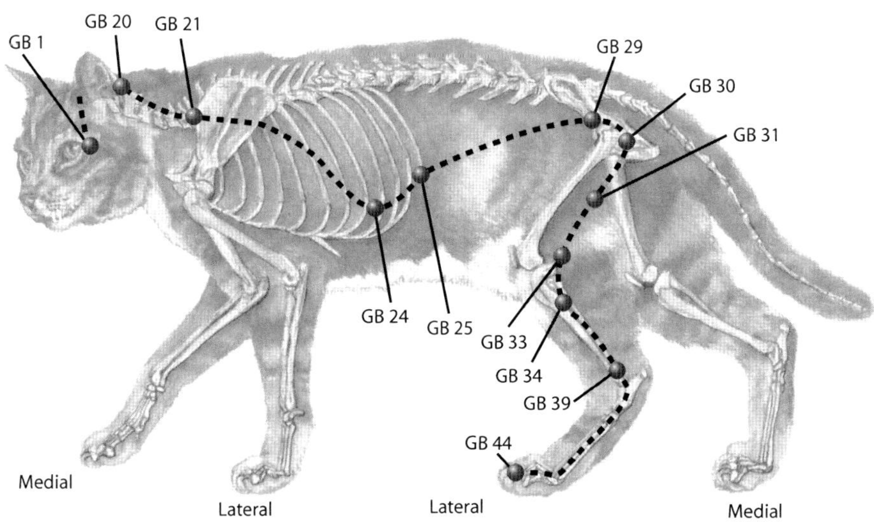

Point	Energetics/Function	Location
GB 1	Brightens eyes, dispels Wind and clears Fire and Heat. **Benefits** ocular disorders and facial paralysis.	In a depression over rim of the orbit, just lateral to outer canthus of the eye.
GB 20	Dispels Wind, subdues Liver-Yang, facilitates chi flow, and clears brain. **Benefits** cervical issues, epilepsy, and eye disorders.	Dorsal aspect of neck, caudal to the occipital bone, and cranial to the wing of the atlas.
GB 21	Spreads Liver chi, removes Liv Wind, facilitates all chi flow, clears Heat. **Benefits** shoulder and back pain, Liv and GB disorders, expedites labor, and facilitates lactation. Contraindicated in pregnancy.	Just cranial to scapula, between the 7th cervical and 1st thoracic vertebrae.

Gall Bladder Meridian

Point	Energetics/Function	Location
GB 24	Alarm pt of GB. Regulates Liv, GB, and Stomach. Spreads Liver chi. **Benefits** shoulder pain, or fatigued extremities. Expels gallstones.	At the 9th intercostal space, just ventral to the costochondral junction.
GB 25	Alarm pt of Ki. Tonifies Ki, warms Yang. **Benefits** abdominal or back pain, water metabolism disorders. Expels urinary tract stones.	Found on the lateral side of the abdomen on the tip of the free end of the 13th rib.
GB 29	Dispels Wind, Cold, and clears Heat. **Benefits** lower back, all hip joint disorders, and osteoarthritis.	At the coxofemoral joint in a depression cranial to the greater trochanter of the femur.
GB 30	Dispels Wind and Cold, clears Heat, transforms dampness. **Benefits** lower back & hips, pelvic limb paresis or paralysis, gluteal muscle pain.	In a depression midway between the greater trochanter of the femur and the tuber ischii.
GB 31	Dispels Wind and Cold, clears Heat. **Benefits** pelvic limb disorders.	Lateral aspect of the thigh, 7 cun above the lateral epicondyle of the femur.
GB 33	Dispels Wind and Cold, clears Heat, transforms Dampness. **Benefits** stifle pain and osteoarthritis.	Lateral side of the pelvic limb at the stifle, in a depression above the lateral epicondyle of the femur.
GB 34	Regulates and tonifies Liv & GB, spreads Liv chi, extinguishes Liv Wind, facilitates chi flow, Influential pt for tendons and ligaments. **Benefits** flow of blood and chi in limbs, hypertension, vomiting, Liver and GB disorders, Stomach and Liver chi stagnation, and general pain relief.	Lateral aspect of the hind limb, in a depression in front of and below the head of the fibula.
GB 40	Source pt. Regulates Liv and GB, spreads Liver chi. **Benefits** lower back, thigh and intercostal pain, vomiting, and hock pain.	On the lateral aspect of the hind limb, directly distal to the lateral malleolus of the fibula.

Gall Bladder Meridian

Point	Energeticcs/Function	Location
GB 41	Regulates Liv, GB, spreads Liver chi, extinguishes Liver Wind. **Benefits** ocular issues, metatarsal pain, irregular cycles, hip pain, and lactation.	In a depression below the junction of the 4th and 5th metatarsal bones.
GB 44	Jing-well pt. Regulates GB, dispels Wind, and clears Heat. **Benefits** febrile issues, hypertension, shock, and ocular disorders.	On the lateral side of the 4th digit of the hind paw, at the nail bed.

Gall Bladder Meridian

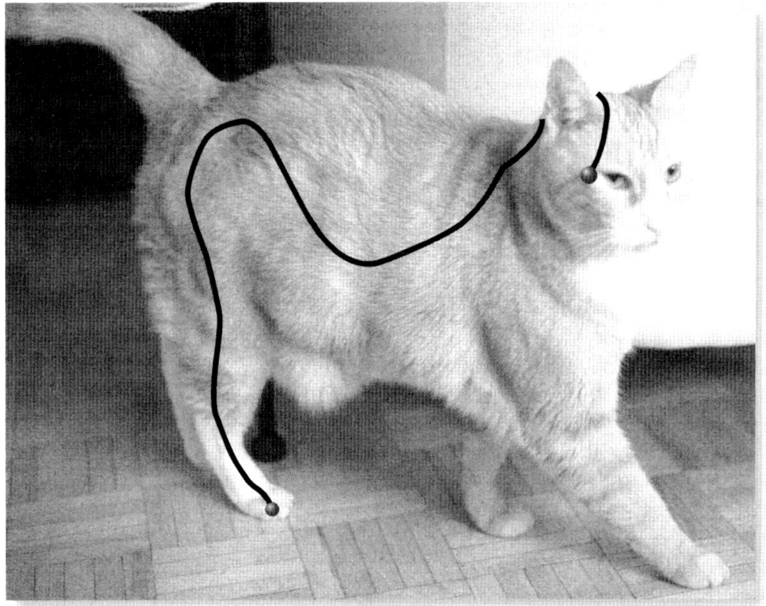

Liver
Hind Leg *Jueyin* / Absolute Yin
Controller of Strategic Planning

The Liver ensures the smooth, harmonious flow of chi throughout the cat's body. The Liver stores and replenishes blood while also managing the volume of blood in response to demand of physical activity. Known as *Gan* in Chinese, the Liver plays a role in the entire body's energetics and nourishment of tissues. It has a significant role in digestion, too. As the Strategic Planner, the Liver is involved in all the body functions, that is, all of the other internal organs are dependent on the proper functioning of the Liver. The Gallbladder is the yang organ system paired with the Liver.

Functions & Attributes

- Governs harmonious flow of chi
- Stores and replenishes blood
- Regulates the volume of blood
- Controls the sinews (tendons and ligaments)
- Manifests in the nails / claws
- Sensory orifice is the eyes
- Fluid is bile
- Emotion is anger
- Belongs to the Wood Element
- Optimal flow of Chi 1 – 3 AM

Health Issues

- Muscle spasms, seizures, convulsions
- Tendon and ligament problems
- Nail or claw issues
- Stiff or cramped muscles
- Vision or eye disorders
- Estrous cycle problems
- Reproductive issues
- Digestive problems
- Joint problems
- Toxic issues
- Low energy
- Blood disorders

Emotional Issues

- Depression
- Lack of initiative
- Aggressiveness or anger
- Chaotic behavior
- Irritability

Location and Flow of the Liver Meridian

The Liver Meridian begins on the hind leg. Liver 1 is on the lateral side of the second digit. The meridian travels up the metatarsals to the hock (ankle) crossing over the joint to the medial aspect of the hind leg, goes past the stifle (knee) joint and up to the inguinal groove (groin area). It then enters the pubic region and travels forward toward the head on the lower third of the rib cage. The next to the last point, Liver 13, is located at the end of the twelfth rib. The Liver meridian then slants downward and ends with Liver 14, at the sixth intercostal space.

Liver Meridian

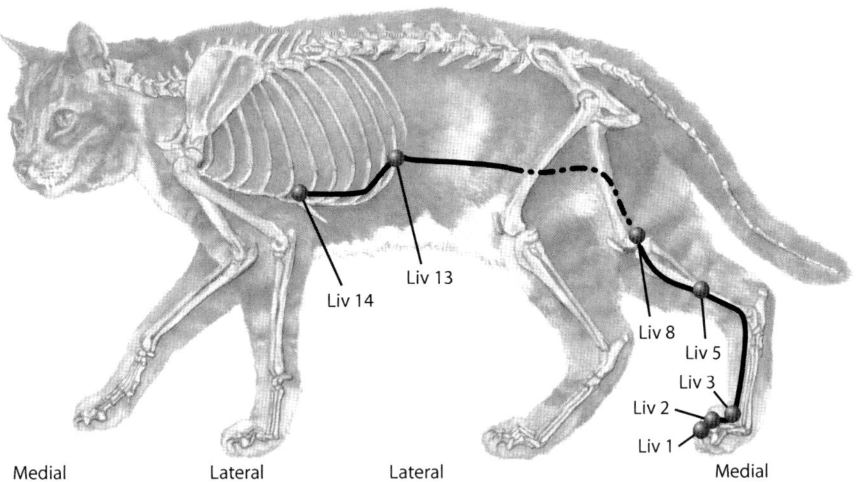

Point	Energetics/Function	Location
Liv 1	Jing-well point. Regulates and tonifies Liver, spreads Liver chi, helps contain blood. **Benefits** urinary incontinence, irregular estrous, and all types of bleeding.	Lateral side of 2nd digit of hind paw, at the nail bed
Liv 2	Regulates Liver, invigorates blood, calms spirit, extinguishes Liver Wind. **Benefits** irregular estrous, ocular issues, seizures, and urinary incontinence or retention.	Distal to the metatarsophalangeal joint, on the lateral side of the 2nd digit.
Liv 3	Source pt, regulates and tonifies Liver invigorates blood, regulates chi. **Benefits** Liver and GB disorders, endocrine and metabolic disorders (diabetes mellitus), distal eye point, hock pain, and toxin removal.	Between the 2nd and 3rd metatarsal bones at the junction of the metatarsophalangeal joint.

Liver Meridian

Point	Energetics/Function	Location
Liv 5	Connecting pt. Regulates and tonifies Liver, spreads Liver chi, enriches Yin and contains blood. **Benefits** impotence, irregular estrous, sterility, muscle spasms of back, or urinary incontinence. Loss of consciousness point.	Medial side of hindleg, caudal to the tibia and cranial to gastrocnemius muscle about 1/4 of the distance from the medial malleolus of tibia to the stifle joint.
Liv 8	Regulates and tonifies Liver, spreads Liver chi, and tonifies the blood. **Benefits** urinary incontinence, male and female reproductive disorders, or stifle pain.	In a depression on the medial end of the transverse popliteal crease, between the medial condyle of femur and the attachment of semimembranosus muscle.
Liv 13	Alarm point for Sp, regulates, tonifies and strengthens Spleen, reduces digestive stagnation, regulates Stomach, warms Cold. Influential point of Yin organs. **Benefits** food stagnation, abdominal masses and pain, fatigued or painful extremities, and harmonizes Liver and Stomach.	On the ventrolateral side of the abdomen at the costochondral junction of 12th rib.
Liv 14	Alarm point for Liver, regulates Liver and GB, spreads Liver chi, expands and relaxes chest. **Benefits** the emotions, Liver and Stomach, hypertension and cirrhosis. Promotes lactation.	In the 6th intercostal space, at the level of the mammary line.

Conception Vessel & Governing Vessel

Ren Mai / *Yin Gathering Vessel* & *Du Mai* / *Yang Gathering Vessel*

There are eight extraordinary vessels, or channels, that serve as storage or reservoirs for chi. Of these eight extraordinary vessels there are two vessels, the Conception and Governing Vessels, which are usually included with the 12 Major Meridians because they have their own powerful acupoints. Though these two channels are not associated with a particular zang-fu organ, nor are they paired with each other, they are instrumental in maintaining the constant dynamic balance of energy in the body. The remaining six extraordinary vessels do not have their own acupoints. The chi of those six vessels is accessed through points on the 12 Major Meridians.

The Conception Vessel, also known as the *Sea of Yin*, acts as a reservoir for yin chi. The other zang-fu organ systems can use the yin chi as needed to balance yang chi. While the Governing Vessel, also called the *Sea of Yang*, is the reservoir of yang chi and serves to balance the yin chi. The Conception Vessel and Governing Vessels are connected to create the continuous flow of yin and yang. The body is constantly balancing yin and yang.

The Conception and the Governing Vessels receive energy from the Kidney and share the essence that is stored in the Kidney. These vessels, like all the extraordinary vessels circulate Nutrient / *Ying* Chi and Original Chi and serve as the connection with the 12 Major Meridians. The extraordinary vessels function at a deeper level than the main channels and profoundly affect the basic constitution of the cat.

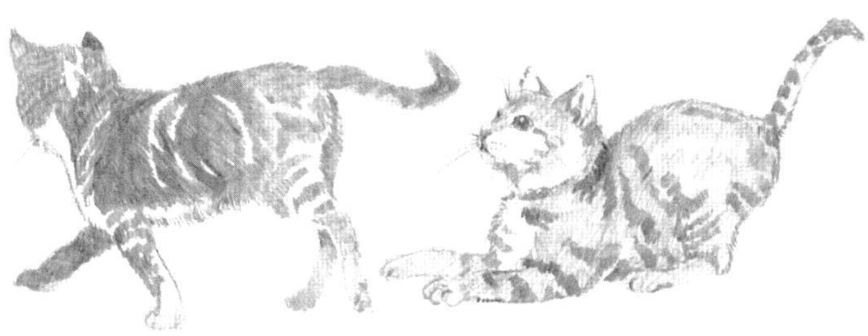

Conception Vessel
Ren Mai
Yin Gathering Vessel

The Conception Vessel absorbs, stores, and transfers yin chi as needed to maintain a dynamic balance within the 12 Major Meridians. The acupoints along this channel have a strong influence on the reproductive system, physical development, and the transportation of chi and blood to the lower compartment of the Triple Heater and the uterus in the female. Additionally, these acupoints can be used to resolve organ issues along the cat's ventral midline. For instance, Conception Vessel 3, Middle Extremity, is located near the Bladder and it is known to benefit urinary problems and enhances the Bladder's capacity to perform chi transformation.

Functions and Attributes

- Unites and balances the 12 Major Meridians
- Nourishes yin chi
- Governs reproduction and fertility
- Governs growth and development
- Governs the peripheral nervous system (outside the spinal column)
- Regulates blood flow in the 12 Major Meridians

Health Issues

- Replenishes Original chi
- Reproductive / fertility issues
- Collapse of yang
- Blood problems
- Digestive issues
- Local pain / disorders

Emotional Issues:

- Hyperactivity
- Anxiety

Location and Flow of the Conception Vessel

The Conception Vessel, called *Du Mai* in Chinese, flows up the ventral midline from just below the perineum, or anus, (Conception Vessel 1) up the abdomen, chest, and throat to a point one cun ventral to the border of the lower lip which is identified as Conception Vessel 24.

Conception Vessel Meridian

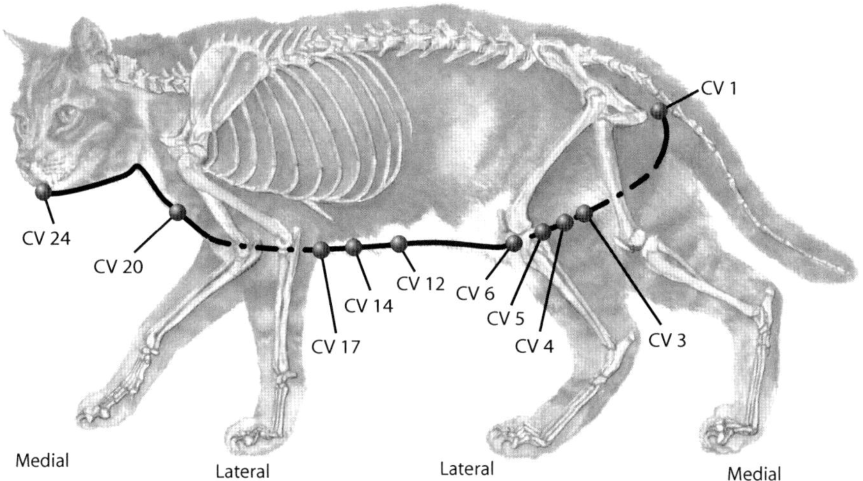

Point	Energetics/Function	Location
CV 1	Stabilizes the Essence, tonifies and regulates chi, revives consciousness and calms the spirit. **Benefits** infertility, uterine prolapse, epilepsy, or colic.	On the ventral midline, halfway between the anus and the scrotum or vulva.
CV 3	Alarm point for Bladder. Regulates the lower burner, clears Heat, and tonifies the Kidneys. **Benefits** incontinence, infertility, renal issues, or impotence.	On the ventral midline, 4 cun caudal to the umbilicus.
CV 4	Alarm point for SI. Tonifies the Kidneys, Source Chi, chi and blood. **Benefits** chi and blood deficiency, general weakness, urine retention, diarrhea, or infertility.	On the ventral midline, 3 cun caudal to the umbilicus.
CV 5	Alarm pt for SI. Tonifies the Kidneys, Source chi, chi and blood. **Benefits** chi and blood deficiency, general weakness, urine retention, diarrhea or infertility.	On the ventral midline, 2 cun caudal to the umbilicus.

Conception Vessel Meridian

Point	Energetics/Function	Location
CV 6	Tonifies the Kidneys, Source chi, regulates the CV, enriches Yin, cools Heat in the blood, calms the fetus. **Benefits** chronic diarrhea, generalized weakness, constipation, abdominal pain. Yang tonic point.	On ventral midline, 1.5 cun caudal to the umbilicus.
CV 12	Alarm point for Stomach, Influential pt for Yang organs. Regulates strengthens and tonifies the Sp, St, and middle burner, tonifies Nutritive chi. **Benefits** gastric ulcers, liver disorders, diarrrhea, vomiting, and generalized weakness.	On ventral midline, halfway between the xiphoid and umbilicus.
CV 14	Alarm point for Heart. Regulates the Heart, calms the spirit, and regulates the chi. **Benefits** cold extremities, anxiety or fear, gastric ulcers, epilepsy, and vomiting.	On the ventral midline, at about the level of the xiphoid process.
CV 17	Alarm point for Pe. Influential point of chi and Sea of chi point. Regulates the Lung, regulates and tonifies chi. **Benefits** cough, vomiting, and facilitates and expedites lactation.	On the ventral midline, at the level of the caudal border of the elbow, 4th intercostal space.
CV 20	Regulates and descends chi. **Benefits** cough, respiratory disorders, and difficult breathing.	Ventral midline at level of 1st intercostal space.
CV 24	Dispels Wind, clears Heat, transforms Dampness and Phlegm. **Benefits** behavioral disorders, mania, seizures, gingivitis, gum, or tooth pain.	Ventral midline, 1 cun ventral to the border of the lower lip.

Conception Vessel Meridian

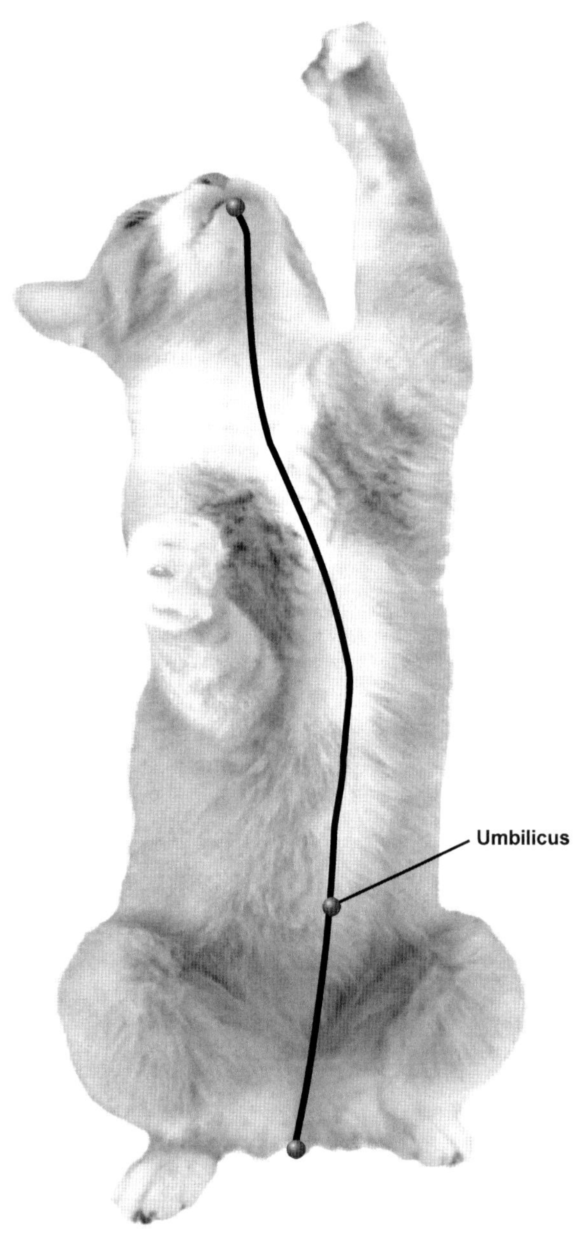

Governing Vessel
Du Mai
Yang Gathering Vessel

The Governing Vessel influences the yang channels and enhances yang chi of the cat's entire body. Other specific attributes of the Governing Vessel include strengthening the spine, nourishing the brain, expelling internal and external wind, and increasing Kidney yang chi. The Governing Vessel acupoints also benefit the local areas and organs along its' pathway. An example of this is Governing Vessel 4, Gate of Vitality (located just above the kidneys), enhances Kidney function and strengthens the lower back.

There are many energetics and functions associated with each of the acupoints on the Governing Vessel. In Chinese this channel is called *Du Mai.* It absorbs, stores, and transfers yang chi in the same way the Conception Vessel serves as a reservoir and distribution system of yin chi for the 12 Major Meridians. The Governing vessel provides the balance of yang chi throughout the meridian system.

Functions and Attributes

- Unites and balances yang chi within the 12 Major Meridians
- Governs the central nervous system
- Governs blood circulation
- Strengthens the spine
- Nourishes marrow and the brain
- Influences organs along the dorsal midline

Health Issues

- Autonomic nervous system issues
- Blood circulation problems
- External or internal invasion of wind
- Spinal pain or soreness
- Unconsciousness
- Respiratory emergency
- Kidney function problem

Emotional Issue

- Anxiety

Location and Flow of the Governing Vessel

The Governing Vessel begins at the depression between the anus and the root of the tail (Governing Vessel 1). The channel travels toward the head along the dorsal midline of the cat's back. It continues over the head, down the center of the muzzle, over the nose, and under the lip to Governing Vessel 28. Governing Vessel 26 is of note since it is commonly used as the consciousness and respiration point in emergencies. Governing Vessel 26 is located on the ventral midline at the lower edge of the cat's nostrils.

Governing Vessel Meridian

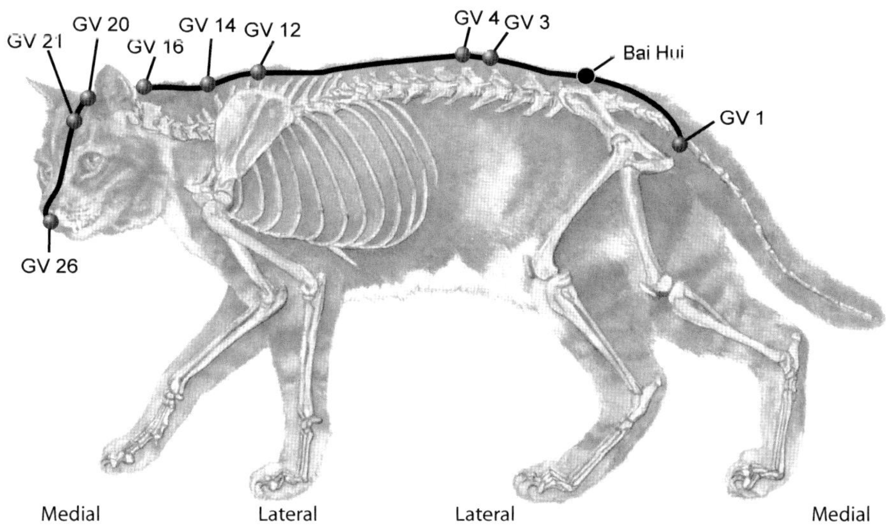

Point	Energetics/Function	Location
GV 1	Connecting point of the GV. Regulates the GV, calms the spirit, and strengthens the lower back. **Benefits** spinal stiffness, lower back pain, seizures, epilepsy, diarrhea, constipation, depression, or fatigue.	On the dorsal midline, in a depression between the anus and the base of the tail.
GV 3	Tonifies chi and Yang of Ki, warms cold. **Benefits** lumbar disc issues, lower back pain, and pelvic limb paralysis.	On dorsal midline, in depression between the spinous processes of the 4th and 5th lumbar vertebrae.
GV 4	Tonifies Kidney chi & Yang, Source chi, and Essence, calms spirit, restores Yang. **Benefits** bone disorders, Yang deficiency, intervertebral disc issues, seizures, infertility, or diarrhea.	On the dorsal midline between the spinous processes of the 2nd and 3rd lumbar vertebrae.
GV 12	Regulates the Lungs, calms the spirit, and clears Heat. **Benefits** shen disturbances, convulsions, cough, upper back stifness and pain.	On dorsal midline in a depression between the 3rd and 4th thoracic vertebrae.

Governing Vessel Meridian

Point	Energetics/Function	Location
GV 14	Sea of Chi Point. Clears Heat, dispels Wind. **Benefits** Yin deficiency, fever, cough, cervical pain, or spondylosis. Strengthens the immune system.	On the dorsal midline between the spinous processes of the 7th cervical and 1st thoracic vertebrae.
GV 16	Clears the brain, opens sensory orifices. **Benefits** intervertebral issues, epilepsy, stroke, blurred vision, hearing, and mania.	On the dorsal midline in a depression between the occipital bones and the1st cervical vertebra.
GV 20	Clears brain, calms the spirit, revives consciousness, spreads Liver chi, dispels Wind, warms and restores collapsed Yang. **Benefits** seizures, shock, neck stiffness, epilepsy, sleep issues, and shen disturbances.	On the dorsal midline level with the front of the ear canal.
GV 21	Clears Heat and the nose, and brightens the eyes. **Benefits** epilepsy, shen disturbances, and hyperactive behavior.	On the dorsal midline at the level of the front edge the ears.
GV 26	Revives consciousness, calms spirit, clears the brain, Heat, and Wind, restores collapsed Yang, regulates the GV, and strengthens the back. **Benefits** emergencies such as shock, collapse, heatstroke, or coma. Helps cervical, thoracic or lumbar disc issues, seizures, or mania.	Located on the vertical line on the upper lip (philtrum) at the level of the lower edge of the nostrils.

Governing Vessel Meridian

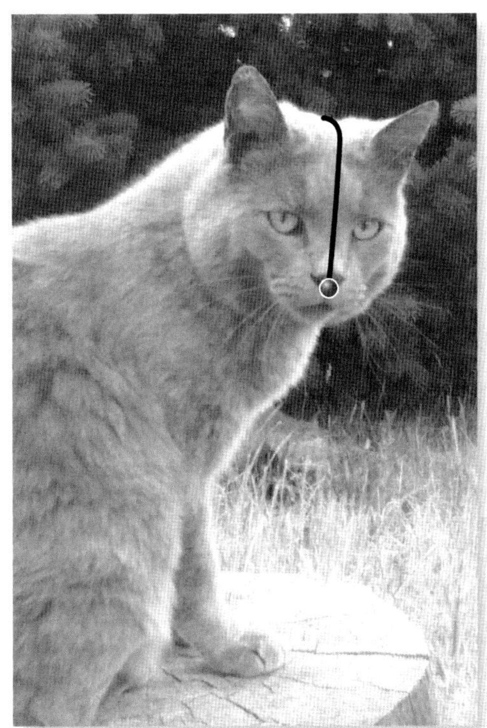

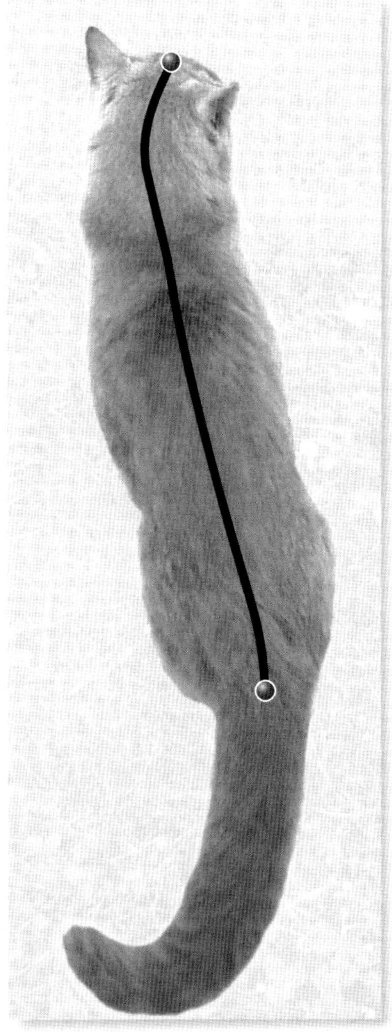

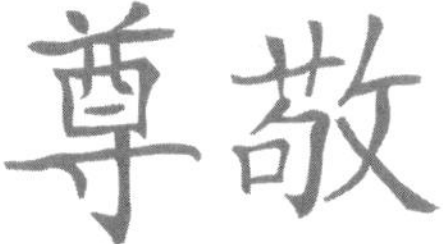

The Use Of Words In Eastern Medicine

Words in eastern medicine carry different meanings than in western conventional medicine. In eastern medicine, referring to "Kidney" evokes a host of energetic information and body functions related to the Kidney channel and the physical kidneys. The implications in Chinese medicine are quite different than in western medicine.

When identifying an imbalance or a pattern of disharmony, be careful not to sound alarms by using words that others may not have the same reference. Saying there's heat along the Bladder Meridian near the kidneys might sound scary to someone who is not familiar with Chinese medicine.

On the other hand, there are times when you will discover an inflammation, injury, or disease pattern that needs veterinary attention. It's important to know when to make the judgment call to visit the veterinarian. If there's even the slightest question your cat should be seen by a vet, be sure to take him. Always have his best interest firmly in mind.

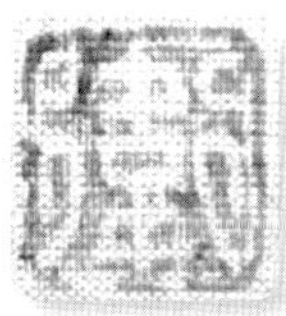

Reference: Cun Measurement

In Chinese medicine, cun measurement is used to locate acupoints. Cun, pronounced "tsun," means "little measurement." A cun measurement is relative and proportional to the conformation of each individual cat. A cun measurement identifies the distance from one anatomical landmark to another or one acupoint to another. Because cats vary in size and conformation, the length of a cun on a Maine Coon is usually going to be larger than on a delicate Siamese. The cun provides a more accurate method of measurement than inches or centimeters because it is specific to a particular cat's body.

There are a number of methods of determining the length of a cun. For an average size cat, you can use the distance from the elbow crease to the cat's carpus (wrist) to determine a cun. For a cat with short legs, use the

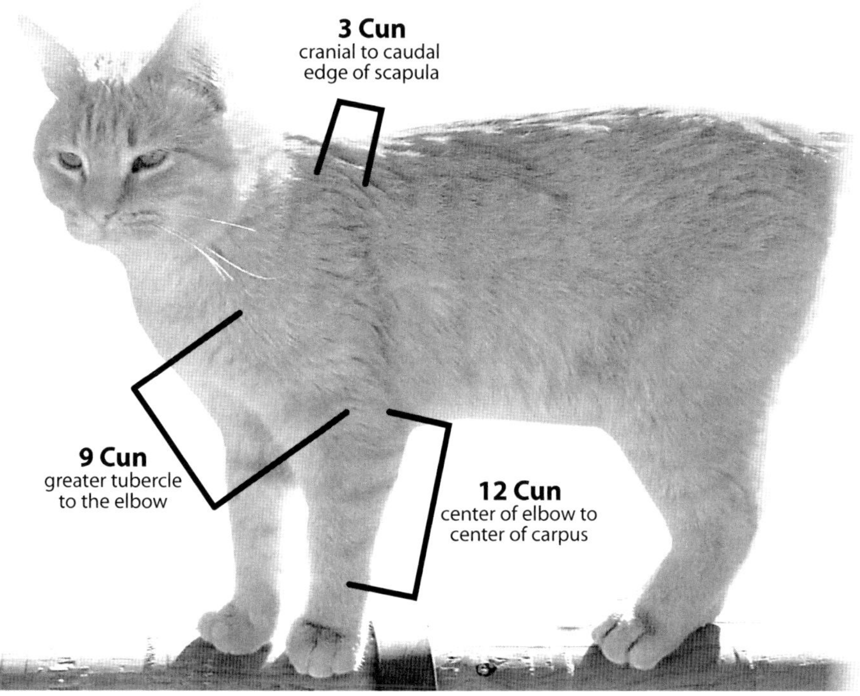

front to the back edge of the scapula (shoulder blade) as your reference to determine the cun measurement. Select the method that best suits your cat.

For example, measure the distance from the shoulder joint to the elbow crease on the front leg. Simply divide that distance into three equal portions and you will be able to measure 3 cun. Compare this to the finger-width of the distance between your pointer finger to your ring finger and note where the 3 cun mark is in relation to the width of your fingers. If you know 3 cun and the location calls for 1 cun, divide the distance by 3 and you will know how to measure 1 cun.

The next example is using the lower segment of your cat's front leg. A cun is 1/12th the distance between the carpus (wrist) and the elbow crease. The cun measurement can be found by dividing the distance in half, then halving the distance on the lower portion again and this yields 3 cun. Using your hand or finger-width you can use this measurement to approximate distances from given anatomical landmarks or other acupoints.

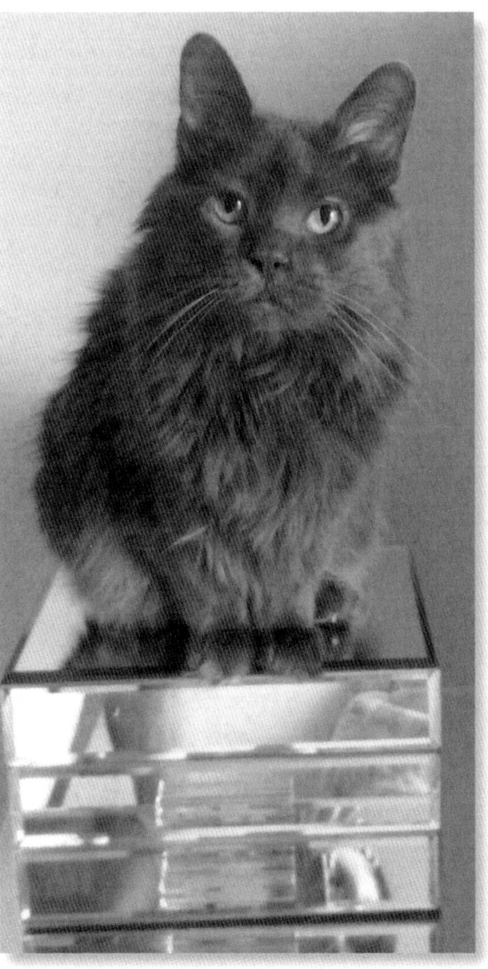

Measuring the top of the scapula from the front edge to the back edge gives you 3 cun. Again, measure that distance against your finger-width and you will be able to apply cun measurement on the cat's body by using your own hand.

Chapter Five

Acupressure Points & Classifications

Just touching our cats puts us in touch with the better part of ourselves. Their gentle souls remind us of who we really are. When caring for their needs, we are caring for our own needs. We can get so caught up in a "cat-rillion" demands, we forget about the simple joys of daily life until our favorite cat catches our attention. The instant we connect with him, our whole being changes. We soften inside and feel an inner contentment by sharing a moment or two with our special feline friend.

Acupressure, human caring, and cats are a good combination for mending both torn people and torn cats. Learning about acupressure points is the next step toward caring for your cats—and yourself—through this work.

"If a man could be crossed with the cat, it would improve the man but deteriorate the cat."
— Mark Twain

Acupoints

In an acupressure session, the purpose of using acupressure points is to resolve imbalances in the zang-fu organ systems (the internal organs and their respective meridians). When there is a blockage along a meridian, stimulating the acupressure point that's known to resolve that type of blockage or energetic imbalance will restore the harmonious flow of chi and blood to the entire body. Any imbalance within the zang-fu organ system means that the cat's body is not functioning optimally and can succumb to illness. Acupressure points are the "tools" of acupressure.

An acupressure point, commonly called an "acupoint," is a specific location along a meridian where chi pools. At these pools of energy, we can stimulate and affect the flow of chi and blood along the meridian. Acupoints are found just under the surface of the skin. They tend to be located on soft tissue rather than on bony prominences or in the belly of a muscle. You'll find them in the depressions next to (or between) muscles and bones and around joints.

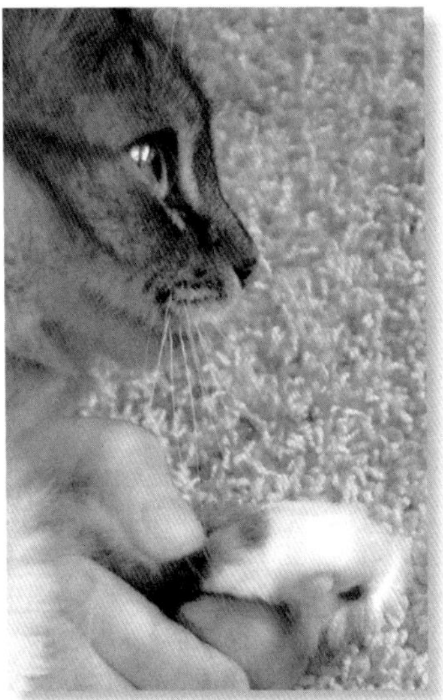
Large Intestine 4

There are 361 known acupoints on the feline body. These points are along the 12 Major Meridians and the two Extraordinary Vessels. Considered permanent acupoints because they exist all the time, they are identified by their functions, locations, and effects on the body.

For instance, the acupoint called "Large Intestine 4" is a specific acupoint located along the Large Intestine meridian. This point is located at your cat's dewclaw. When you hold or stimulate Large Intestine 4, your cat may experience the energetic and functional benefits of this point. Because this point is sedating, your cat may feel more relaxed. If he has any sinus congestion, pressing this point can help drain his sinuses.

Large Intestine 4 can reduce fever and promote a healthy level of moisture in the skin. This point is known to aid in dental, jaw, shoulder, elbow, and carpus (wrist) issues because of the meridian's location flowing through the lower part of the forelimb. Like Large Intestine 4, each of the known acupoints has its own properties.

Another example is Heart 7 located on the Heart meridian. This acupoint is commonly used to support the heart's role in circulating blood through the vascular system. Other properties of Heart 7 include the following: cools heat in the blood, calms the spirit, strengthens and clears the brain. Heart 7 is used to dispel mania, seizures, depression, hyperactivity, anxiety, and other behavioral problems. Clearly, Heart 7, like many acupoints, is a powerful point.

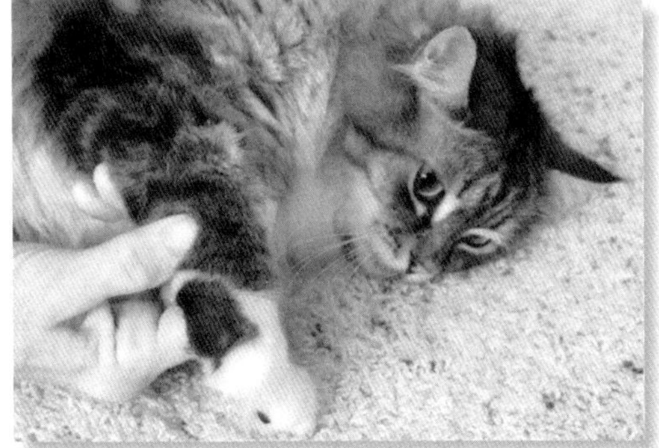
Heart 7

There are acupoints that are not located along a meridian

or vessel. These points are considered interim points, or *Ah Shi* points, and they only become apparent during states of tension, injury, or illness. These points usually present as hard spots within a muscle. Be careful; they can be painful and your cat will probably exhibit a jump reaction or something more adverse when you touch one of these points. Be gentle with your touch.

Acupoint Classifications

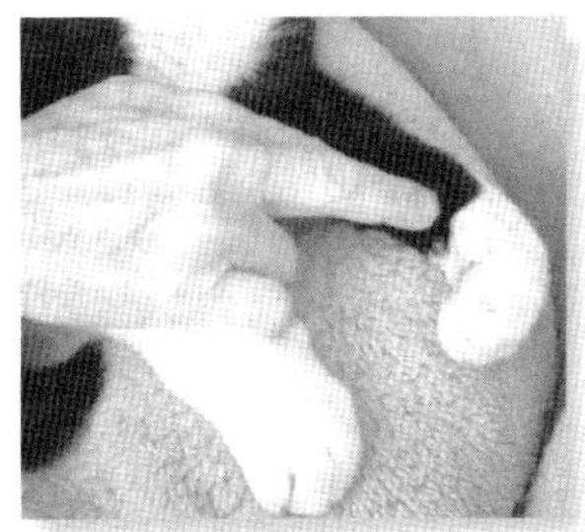
Lung 7

Over thousands of years of clinical observation, practitioners have noted acupoints that have specific energetics and functions in common. These acupoints have been placed into categories for ease of use. Acupoint classifications are the "medicine bag" of the TCM practitioner.

Acupoints are classified or grouped by how they benefit the body. For example, Master points benefit specific regions of the body. They are used to enhance an acupressure session that's intended to resolve an issue related to a particular area of the body. Lung 7 is the Master point for the head and neck. When your cat has sinus, eye, ear, jaw, or neck issues, you can add Lung 7 to your acupressure session.

Bladder 40 is the Master point that benefits the hindquarters. You can stimulate Bladder 40 when your cat presents with any disease, pain, or restricted movement related to the lower back, hips, stifle (knee), or hock (ankle). Bladder 40 benefits the hindquarters the way Lung 7 benefits the head and neck; they are both Master points. When included in a session, you'll find that Master points enhance the effectiveness of the other acupoints selected to deal with an issue in a particular anatomical region.

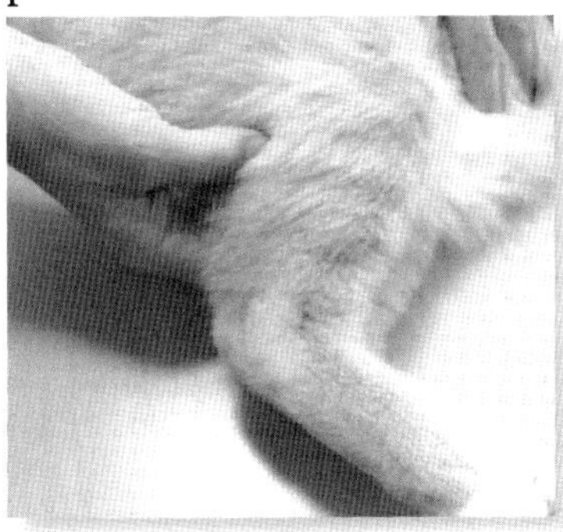
Bladder 40

There are many acupoint classifications. Those covered here include: Association, Alarm, Source, Master, Influential, and Jing-Well points. Each of these classifications is described in this chapter. Having knowledge of these groupings is especially handy in a session with your cat because working one specific point may be all he needs to go on his merry way.

Association Points

Association points, also called Back *Shu* points, are directly connected to the internal organ for which it is named. The Association points are located on the inner channel of the Bladder meridian that is on the dorsal aspect of the cat. These points convey the energy of one of the 12 major zang-fu organ systems. Bladder 13, for example, is the Association point for the Lung. Notice that Bladder 13 is located directly above the Lung organ. Bladder 15 is the Association point for the Heart. Notice this point is above the Heart organ.

Association points help assess the cat's condition and can be used during your acupressure session as well. When touching Bladder 13, you can feel if there's an imbalance within the Lung organ system. If the point feels hotter or warmer than the rest of the cat's body, you will know that an imbalance exists. If the cat reacts or the point feels cool, you can suspect an imbalance in the Lung organ system.

When you detect a Lung imbalance, you can select Bladder 13 for your Point Work during the acupressure session. It has a direct energetic connection with the Lung and thus a strong balancing effect on the Lung. If your cat has a drippy nose or respiratory congestion, Bladder 13 is a good point to stimulate to resolve these issues as part of your session protocol.

Say your cat has digestion issues. Bladder 20 is the Association point for the Spleen while Bladder 21 is the Association point for the Stomach. In TCM, both the Spleen and Stomach are involved in the digestive process. Even if you don't feel any definitive difference in temperature or texture of these two acupoints during your assessment, using Bladder 20 and Bladder 21 in an acupressure session can balance these organ systems and ease digestive problems.

Association points are particularly good in working with cats because they are located along the Bladder meridian, which is approximately ½ to 1½ finger widths away from the dorsal midline (spine), lateral to the spinous processes. Relatively noninvasive, these points are located where cats usually like to be petted.

Association Points

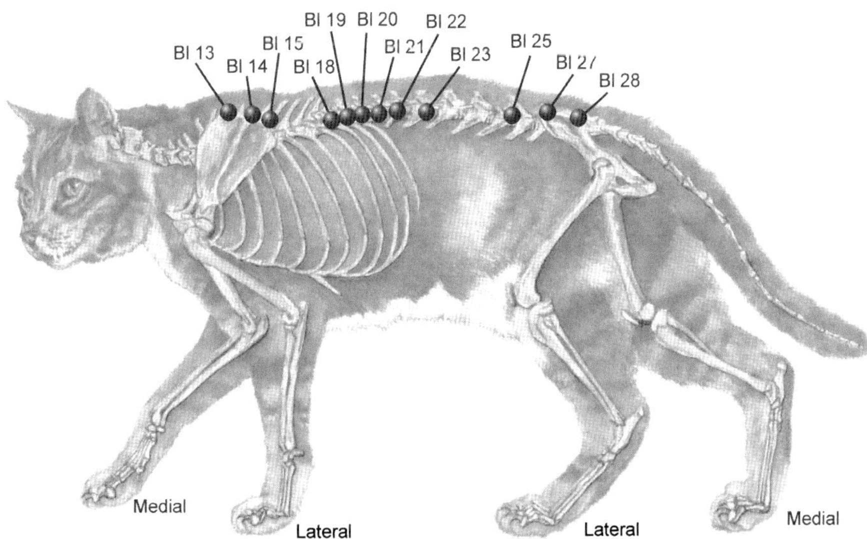

Point	Meridian – Location
Bl 13	Lung –1.5 cun lateral to back edge of dorsal spinous process of 3rd thoracic vertebra.
Bl 14	Pericardium – 1.5 cun lateral to back edge of dorsal spinous process of 4th thoracic vertebra.
Bl 15	Heart –1.5 cun lateral to back edge of dorsal spinous process of 5th thoracic vertebra.
Bl 18	Liver – 1.5 cun lateral to back edge of dorsal spinous process of 10th thoracic vertebra.
Bl 19	Gall Bladder – 1.5 cun lateral to back edge of dorsal spinous process of 11th thoracic vertebra.
Bl 20	Spleen – 1.5 cun lateral to back edge of dorsal spinous process of 12th thoracic vertebra.
Bl 21	Stomach – 1.5 cun lateral to back edge of dorsal spinous process of 13th thoracic vertebra.
Bl 22	Triple Heater – 1.5 cun lateral to back edge of dorsal spinous process of 1st lumbar vertebra.
Bl 23	Kidney – 1.5 cun lateral to back edge of dorsal spinous process of 2nd lumbar vertebra.
Bl 25	Large Intestine – 1.5 cun lateral to back edge of dorsal spinous process of 5th lumbar vertebra.
Bl 27	Small Intestine – 1.5 cun lateral to back edge of dorsal spinous process of 7th lumbar vertebra.
Bl 28	Bladder – Located lateral to 2nd foramen, in depression between sacrum and medial border of dorsal iliac spine.

Alarm Points

Alarm points, also called Front *Mu* Points, are where chi of the zang-fu organ gathers when there's an imbalance or the organ cannot function properly due to illness. Each of the 12 Major organ systems is directly connected to an Alarm point.

Alarm points are used to assess the cat's conditions. They can alert you to any organ involvement rather than simply a meridian imbalance. An organ imbalance or illness is deeper than a meridian imbalance. Meridians are relatively superficial because they travel just beneath the skin. In acupressure, we want to manage health issues at the meridian level. However, there are times when the organ function is disrupted and the chi energy of the organ accumulates in an Alarm point.

All 12 of the Alarm points are located on the ventral or ventrolateral aspect of the cat's trunk. These points can be tender to the touch and need to be approached very lightly. You'll know by the cat's reaction when an Alarm point is tender. You will also know that the organ related to that point needs attention.

Alarm points can be used during the assessment phase and the Point Work segment of your acupressure session. They are often used in combination with Association points.

For example, you have noticed that your cat, Slugger, is constipated. While checking the Association point for Bladder 25, you also notice the Association point for the Large Intestine feels soft, cool, and indented. When you gently check the Alarm point for Large Intestine, Stomach 25, Slugger squirms away from you, indicating the point hurts. In your next acupressure session with Slugger, you can gingerly palpate both Bladder 25 and Stomach 25 to allow the Large Intestine organ to regain a balanced flow of chi and blood.

Alarm Points

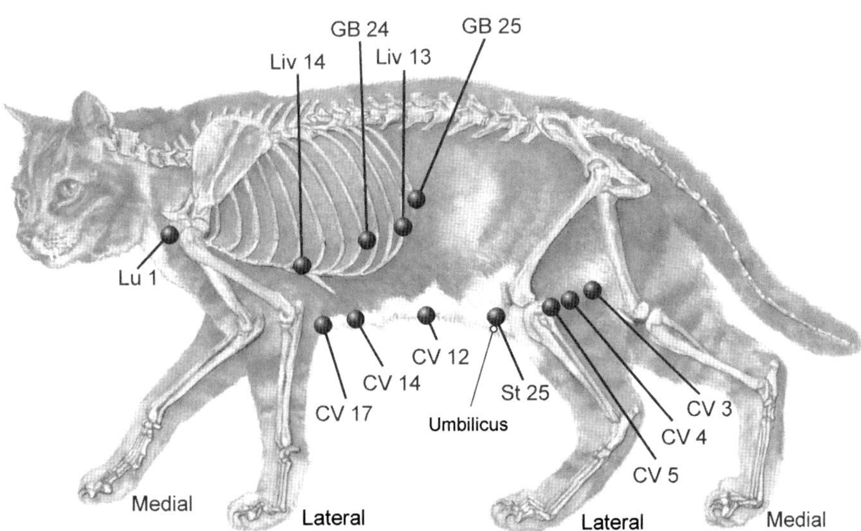

Point	Location
Lu 1	Located at the level of the 1st intercostal space, medial to the greater tubercle of the humerus, in the pectoral muscle. **Alarm point for Lung.**
St 25	2 cun lateral to center of the umbilicus. **Alarm point for Large Intestine.**
CV 12	Located on the ventral midline, halfway between the xiphoid process and the umbilicus. **Alarm point for Stomach.**
Liv 13	On the ventrolateral side of the abdomen at the costochondral junction of the 12th rib. **Alarm point for Spleen.**
CV 14	Ventral midline, at the level of xiphoid process. **Alarm point for Heart.**
CV 4	Ventral midline, 3 cun caudal to umbilicus. **Alarm point for Small Intestine.**
CV 3	Located on the ventral midline, 4 cun caudal to the umbilicus. **Alarm point for Bladder.**
GB 25	Found on the lateral side of the abdomen on the tip of the free end of the 13th rib. **Alarm point for Kidney.**
CV 17	On the ventral midline, at the level of the caudal border of the elbow. **Alarm point for Pericardium.**
CV 5	Ventral midline, 2 cun caudal to umbilicus. **Alarm point for Triple Heater.**
GB 24	At 9th intercostal space slightly ventral to the costochondral junction. **Alarm point for Gall Bladder.**
Liv 14	In the 6th intercostal space, at the level of the mammary line. **Alarm point for Liver.**

Source Points

Source points, or *Yuan* points, are where original or source chi can be accessed. Each of the 12 Major Meridians has a Source point located around the carpus (wrist) on the foreleg and the hock (ankle) on the hind leg. The Triple Heater meridian is responsible for taking the original essence chi from the Kidney and bringing it to each meridian.

When palpated, Source points bring original chi to the meridian and its associated zang-fu organ. These powerful points have the attribute of responding to the needs of the cat's body at that moment in time. They can restore balance to the entire organ system.

Source points are used for assessment and Point Work during a session. When a Source point is hot and protruding, you'll know there's an excess of chi along the meridian. If a Source point feels cold and lifeless, the meridian is probably lacking chi and is deficient in nature. Either way, holding the point during the Point Work section of your acupressure session will help restore the proper balance to the meridian and thus the organ as well.

Source points are known to be effective in strengthening the yin organs. By palpating the hind limb yin Source points (Kidney 3, Spleen 3, and Liver 3), you are nourishing all of the yin organs throughout the cat's body.

When used in the same session, Association points and Source points yield highly effective Point Work. The Association points provide a direct connection to the zang-fu organ system and the Source points provide the nourishment of original chi.

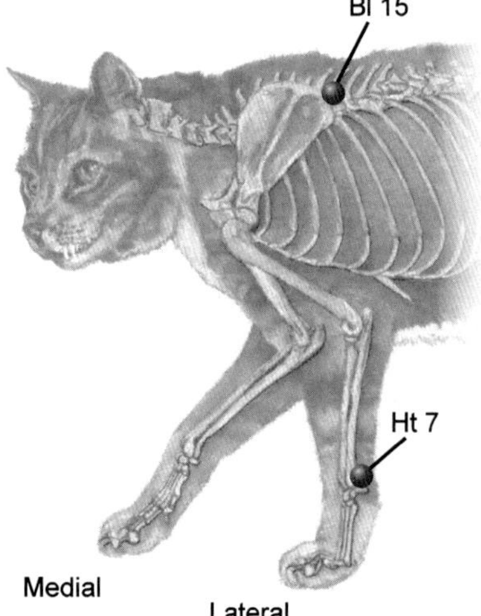

Dixy, a petite British short hair, has exhibited anxiety by constantly hiding under the bed for the past week. "Working" bilaterally (both sides of the cat) Heart 7, the Source point for the Heart, and Bladder 15, the Association point for the Heart—can help reduce Dixy's anxiety reaction. These points address her Heart issue in a direct manner.

Source Points

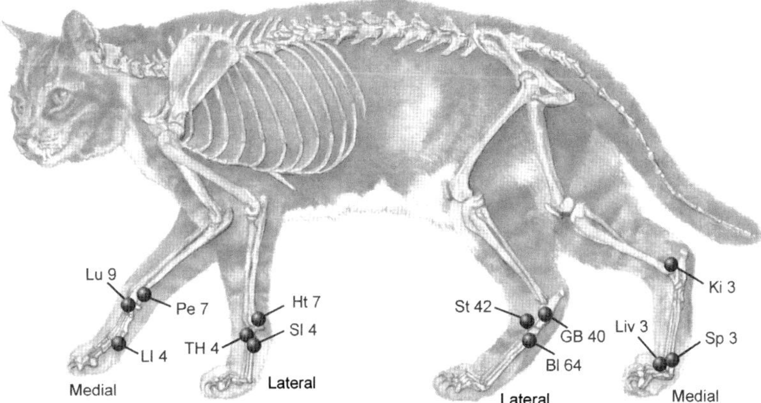

Point	Location
Lu 9	Located on the medial aspect of the radiocarpal joint, just cranial to the radial artery, at the level of Ht 7.
LI 4	Between the first (dewclaw) and 2nd metacarpal bones, on the medial side of the 2nd metacarpal.
St 42	On dorsal aspect of the tarsal joint, at the junction of the 3rd and 4th tarsal bones and the base of the 3rd and 4th metatarsal bones.
Sp 3	Medial aspect of hind leg above metatarsophalangeal joint on the medial side of the 2nd metacarpal bone.
Ht 7	At the transverse crease of the carpal joint, in a depression lateral to the flexor carpi ulnaris. Opposite to Pe 7.
SI 4	Lateral aspect of thoracic limb, below carpal joint, at base of the 5th metacarpal bone.
Bl 64	Located on the lateral aspect of the hind leg, in a depression below and behind the tuberosity of the 5th metatarsal bone.
Ki 3	In the depression between the medial malleolus of the tibia and the calcaneal tendon. Opposite Bl 60.
Pe 7	Found caudal to the tendon of the flexor carpi radialis and directly above the carpal bone.
TH 4	On the lateral side of the forelimb, at the radiocarpal joint, cranial to the tendon of the common digital extensor.
GB 40	On the lateral aspect of the hind limb, on either side of the lateral malleolus of the fibula.
Liv 3	Between the 2nd and 3rd metatarsal bones at the junction of the metatarsophalangeal joint.

Master Points

There are six Master points located near the carpus of the foreleg and the stifle on the hind leg. Master points can increase the effectiveness of a session in which you find an issue in a specific anatomical region of the body.

Large Intestine 4 is the Master point for the face and mouth. If your cat has any issue related to his face or mouth—e.g., a dental problem, TMJ issue, injured tongue, sinus infection— Large Intestine 4 can be used during Point Work to enhance the balancing effect of the other acupoints you select.

Pericardium 6 is the Master point for the chest and front portion of the abdomen. If your cat is injured in this area, or your female cat has difficulty with lactation, Pericardium 6 will help alleviate these health problems along with other acupoints included in the session.

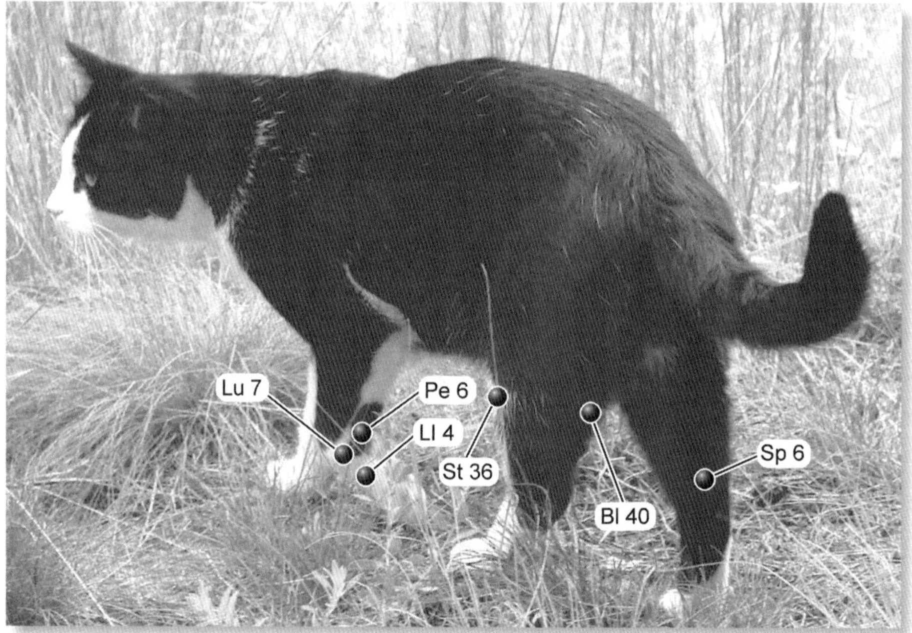

Master Points

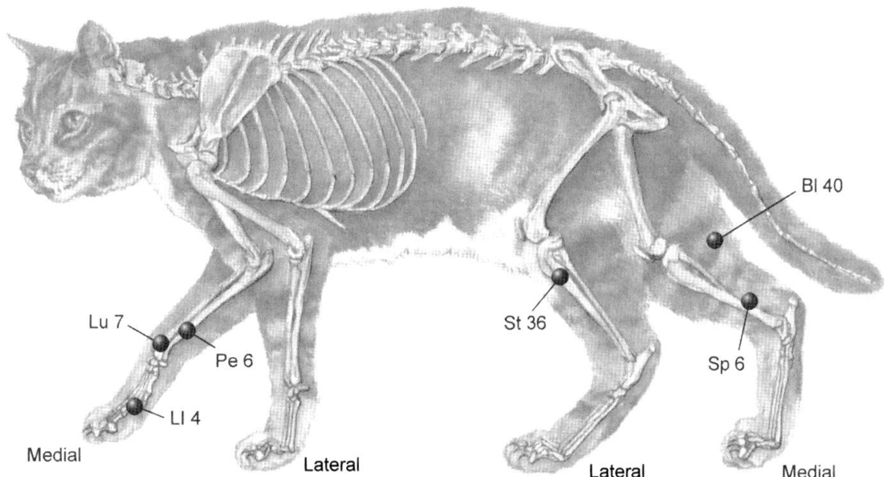

Point	Location
Lu 7	Proximal to the styloid process on radius, 1.5 cun above the transverse crease of the carpus. **Master point for head and neck.**
LI 4	Between the 1st (dewclaw) and 2nd metacarpal bones, on the medial side of the 2nd metacarpal. **Master point for face and mouth.**
St 36	Craniolateral aspect of the pelvic limb. One finger-breadth lateral to the tibial crest, in the lateral portion of the cranial tibial muscle. **Master point for the abdomen and gastrointestinal tract.**
Sp 6	3 cun above tip of medial malleolus on caudal border of tibia. **Master point for the urogenital system and rear portion of abdomen.**
Bl 40	Located at the midpoint of the transverse crease of the popliteal fossa. **Master point for back and hips.**
Pe 6	2 cun above transverse crease of carpus, between tendons of superficial digital flexors. **Master point for chest and front portion of abdomen.**

Influential Points

Influential points, or *Hui* points, have a powerful effect on tissues and functional systems of the body. The 10 Influential points positively impact an acupressure session dealing with the injury or disease of tissues such as bone or tendons and ligaments. They can also positively affect a functional system such as the respiratory system.

Say your cat injures a tendon in his foreleg and is limping. You can use Gall Bladder 34—along with local acupoints above and below the actual injury—to bring more chi and blood to the foreleg and heal the tendon more readily.

You can work Influential points with an older cat that has a long-standing arthritic condition resulting in bone degeneration. Influential points for arthritis are:

- Bladder 11 – Influential point for Bone
- Gall Bladder 39 – Influential point for Marrow

By adding these points to a session you are increasing the flow of chi and blood to the tissue or functional system that is impaired.

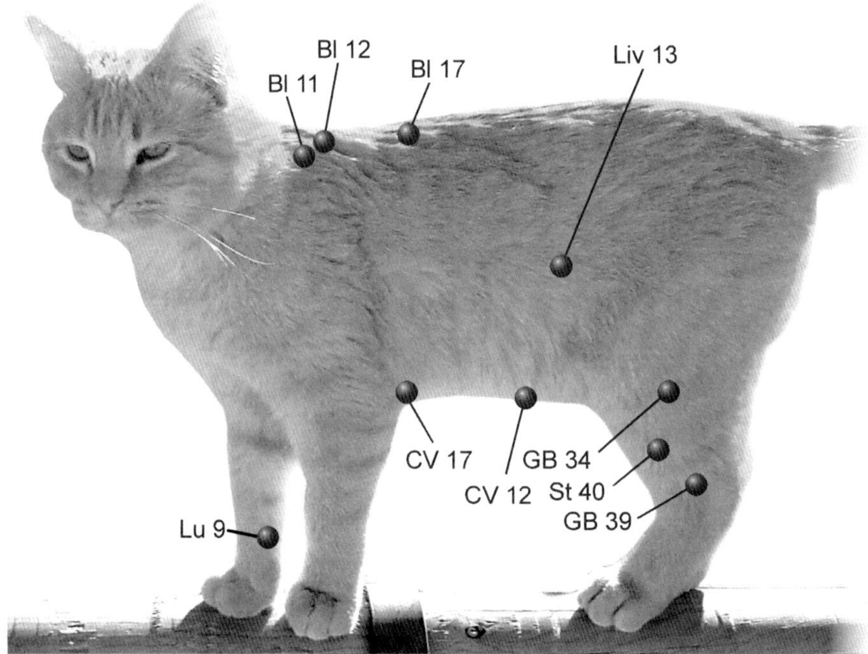

Influential Points

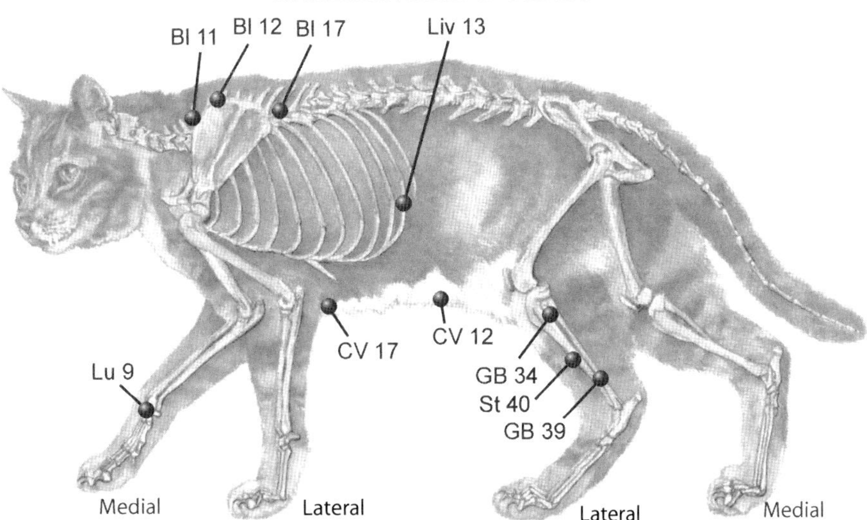

Point	Location
Lu 9	Medial aspect of the radiocarpal joint just cranial to the radial artery, at the level of Ht 7. **Influential point for Arteries.**
St 40	Halfway between lateral malleolus of the fibula and top of the tibia, on the lateral aspect of the pelvic limb. **Influential point for Phlegm.**
BL 11	1.5 cun lateral to caudal border of the spinous process of the 1st thoracic vertebra, at cranial edge of scapula. **Influential point for Bones.**
Bl 12	1.5 cun lateral to the caudal border of the spinous process of the 2nd thoracic vertebra. **Influential point for Wind and Trachea.**
Bl 17	1.5 cun lateral to the caudal border of the spinous process of the 7th thoracic vertebra. **Influential point for Blood and Diaphragm.**
GB 34	Lateral aspect of hind limb, in depression in front of and below the head of the fibula. **Influential point for Tendons and Ligaments.**
GB 39	3 cun above the tip of lateral malleolus, in depression across from Sp 6. **Influential point for Marrow**.
Liv 13	Ventrolateral side of abdomen at the costochondral junction of 12th rib. **Influential point for Yin diseases.**
CV 12	Located on the ventral midline, halfway between the xiphoid process and the umbilicus. **Influential point for Yang diseases**
CV 17	Ventral midline, at the level of caudal border of elbow at the 4th intercostal space. **Influential point for Chi and Respiratory system.**

Jing-Well Points

It is at the *Jing*-Well points where the chi "bubbles up" to the surface. This is where the energy of the 12 Major Meridians transforms from Yin to Yang and Yang to Yin. These points are located at the nail beds, or soft tissue around the claws, and the back of the big pads of the cat's paws. The chi is highly accessible at these points. Jing-well points have the attributes of balancing the entire meridian on which they are located.

The Jing-well points are often used as emergency points and are directly related to the general functions of a meridian. They're known to eliminate pathogenic factors such as fire or cold while harmonizing excess conditions. These points are commonly used to resolve acute conditions like seizures, restoring consciousness, and calming the spirit (*shen*). Jing-well points can be used for both assessment and point work purposes.

Say the cat is experiencing an acute heart issue, Heart 9 or Pericardium 9 can balance the Heart organ system. Liver 1, on the hind paw, can be used during a seizure. Lung 11, the last point on the Lung meridian located on the front paw, is a good point to use when there's a respiratory problem.

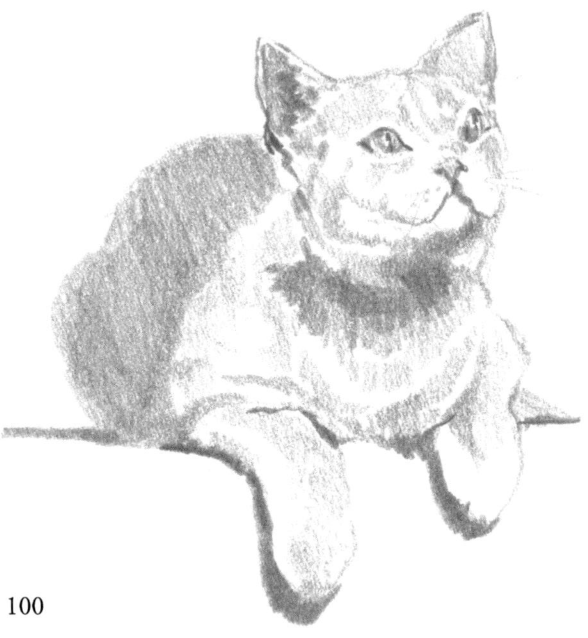

Jing-Well Points

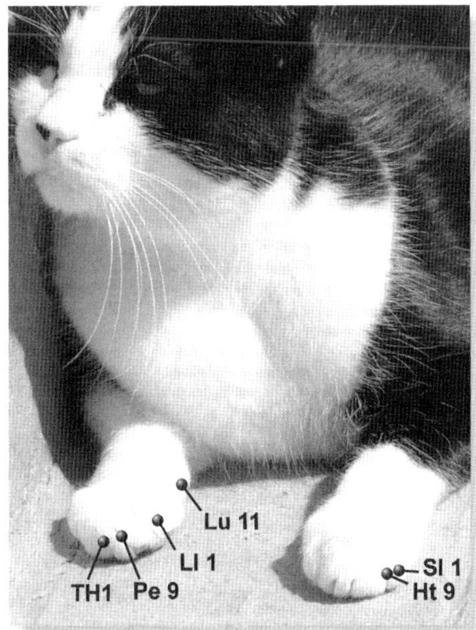

Jing-Well points of the forelegs

Point	Location
Lu 11	Medial side of the dewclaw (digit 1) of the front paw at the nail bed.
LI 1	Medial side of the 2nd digit of the front paw at the nail bed.
Pe 9	Lateral side of the 3rd digit of the front paw at the nail bed.
TH 1	Lateral side of the 4th digit of the front paw at the nail bed.
Ht 9	Medial side of the 5th digit of the front paw at the nail bed.
SI 1	Lateral side of the 5th digit of the front paw at nail bed.

Point	Location
Bl 67	Lateral side of the 5th digit of the hind paw at the nail bed.
Ki 1	Plantar surface of hind paw, at the caudal edge of the metatarsal footpad.
St 45	Lateral side of the 3rd digit of the hind paw at the nail bed.
Sp 1	Medial side of the 2nd digit of the hind paw at the nail bed.
GB 44	On the lateral side of the 4th digit of the hind paw at the nail bed.
Liv 1	Lateral side of 2nd digit of hind paw at the nail bed.

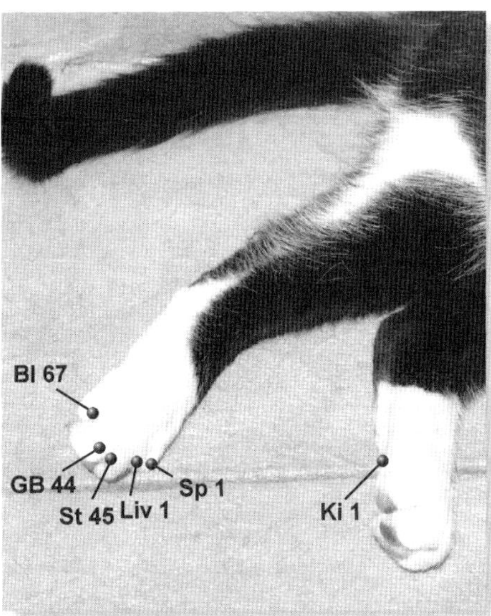

Jing-Well points of the hind legs

I believe cats to be spirits come to earth. A cat, I am sure, could walk on a cloud without coming through.

– Jules Verne

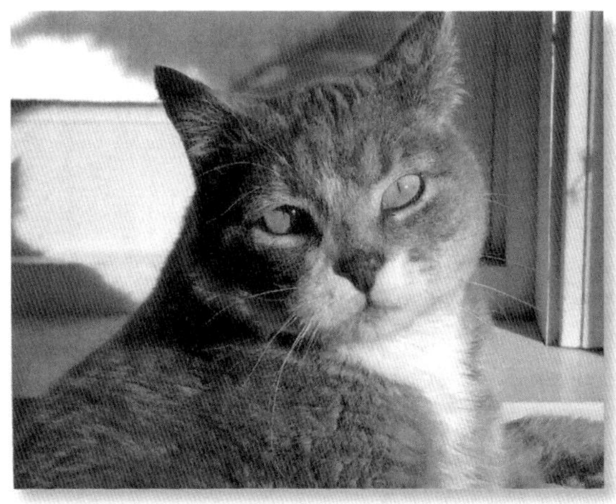

Chapter Six

Assessing Your Cat

Cats can be secretive about how they feel until what's ailing them encroaches on their eating, sleeping, jumping, or running. Your cat has to be feeling poorly when he assumes the "sick-cat position"— crouched down with hind legs tucked under his body, front legs tucked under, too, with the paws sticking out in front under the chest, head held upright and steady with eyes either closed or at half mast. He is keeping all of his energy in and hoping for a healthy outcome.

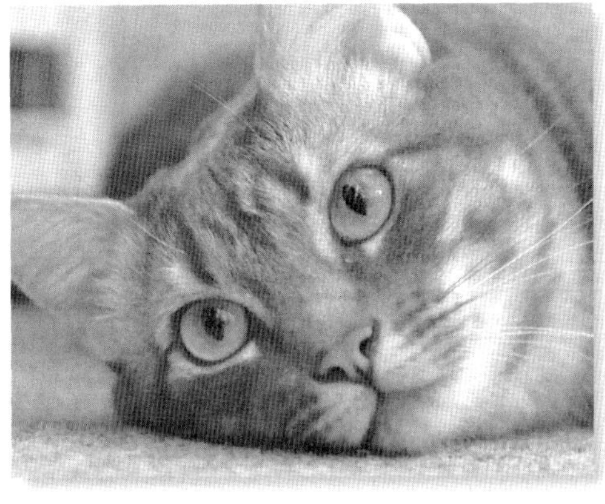

In Traditional Chinese Medicine (TCM), we hope to catch illness before it gets to this state: a cat needing to be in the sick-cat position. Weekly maintenance sessions can help avoid a pattern of imbalance that leads to the cat becoming ill. When the harmonious flow of chi and blood are disrupted, a blockage or stagnation along the meridians can occur. This creates an imbalance within the meridian system that can affect organ function.

By performing an acupressure maintenance session every five to seven days, you're doing your best to resolve imbalances at the meridian level before they can travel more deeply and affect the organs. This will do your cat a world of good and provide for a long and healthy life.

However, things happen, and not always what we want to happen. Cats do get injured. They do get sick. Sometimes, it isn't clear exactly what's going on with your cat. You simply know that he isn't quite right.

With an acute illness, injury, or any kind of health crisis, your holistic veterinarian is your first line of defense. Have your cat checked by a trusted healthcare professional before offering acupressure unless you are using acupoints that are specific emergency points on your way to the veterinary clinic.

Western medicine has excellent trauma care, sophisticated diagnostic tools, and surgical procedures that can save your cat's life. It's an important part of healthcare and, when used in conjunction with Chinese medicine, can give your cat the best of both worlds.

TCM best serves your cat as a way to prevent disease and for chronic health issues. Once you have followed your vet's recommendations and acupressure is not contraindicated, you can proceed to use acupressure. It will restore your cat's balance so he can heal.

The Four Examinations

The Four Examinations, *Se-Zhen*, is a diagnostic technique in which you have to use your senses. The ancient Chinese medical practitioners honed their five senses so they could assess human and animal conditions.

Today, The Four Examinations, also called "The Four Pillars," rely on the practitioner's keen awareness of visible, auditory, olfactory, and touch indicators.

The Four Examinations include:

1. Observation
2. Listening and Smelling
3. Questions / Inquiry
4. Physical Palpation

1. Observation

According to TCM, observation is God-like because it uses one's educated observation skills to see beyond the surface of the body. The ancient Chinese realized that internal issues are manifested externally. It's called the "Law of Integrity." When a stagnation of chi, blood, or body fluids goes on inside the cat and the organs can't function optimally, this can be seen on the outside of the cat's body by educated eyes.

For instance, when your cat has a discharge from his eyes, you will know his Liver needs to be balanced. Why? The Liver is responsible for the health of the eyes. When the Liver is functioning properly, the eyes are bright and healthy. But when the Liver is diseased, the whites of the eyes can turn yellow, showing the presence of jaundice.

"We know the condition of someone's internal organs and the place where the disease exists by observing the external manifestation"

—"Treatise on the Original Organs" from *Miraculous Pivot*

As humans, we tend to look at a cat and know how he is feeling. If your feline is moving slowly and sleeping more than usual, if his eyes appear dull and he isn't grooming himself meticulously, you know he's not feeling well. We are good observers. But then we need to ask, "Is he acting this way because he is emotionally depressed or because of a physical issue? What's not working?" We have to figure out what's going on inside for these external manifestations to exist.

During the observation phase of The Four Examinations, you're looking for your cat's level of vitality, which is evident in the bounce of his step and the brightness of his eyes. Is his weight good? Does he have a discharge from any orifice? Are his teeth clean and white? Are his claws strong and pointed? Any obvious wounds? Is his coat even and clean?

Watching your cat while he grooms himself gives you a good idea of how flexible he is. If he can't reach his entire body, that might indicate his spine needs attention. This may be indicated by an oily or dusty strip down the center of his back.

In Chinese medicine, observing the tongue provides a lot of information about the internal health of the animal. It takes years of conscientious study to know how to interpret the subtleties of distinguishing patterns based on the color, shape, and coatings on the tongue. As an introduction to tongue observation, know that a red tongue indicates a heat imbalance and a pale tongue is evidence of a cold imbalance.

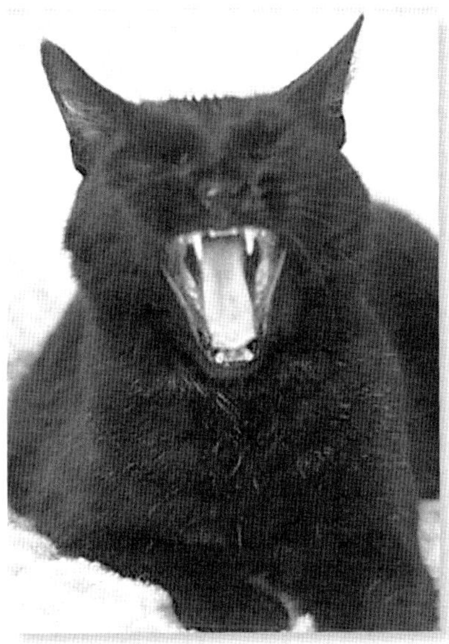

It is important to note the time of day your cat demonstrates discomfort or unhappiness. Chi cycles to each zang-fu organ system through the meridians every 24 hours. Each organ system receives its optimal chi for two hours in succession throughout the 24 hours. These systems receive a "tune up" or extra infusion of chi during the two hours of that period. The cycle begins with the Lung because the first thing a newborn kitten does on its own is breathe its own little breath. The time of Lung is 3 AM to 5 AM.

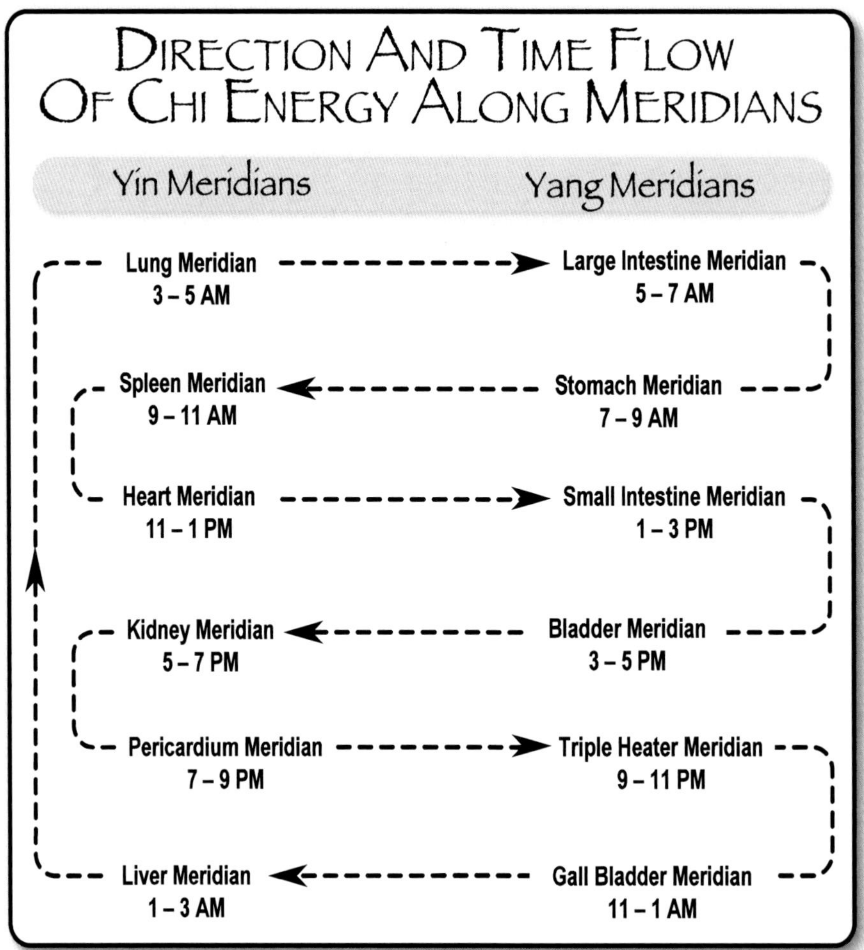

Here's an example of how to use the 24-hour chi-flow clock. Say your house sitter informs you your cat has awakened every morning at 4 AM for the past three days and meows mournfully for an hour or so. You have been away for almost a week and now you know your cat misses you. He's experiencing grief. The time of Lung is 3 to 5 AM and the emotion associated with the Lung is grief and loss. Must be time to go home and give your cat an acupressure session to support his Lung organ system.

Here's another example of using the 24-hour chi flow chart to observe an imbalance in a specific zang-fu organ system. Say your cat is very restless and agitated at about 1:45 PM. He could be indicating that his Small Intestine is not functioning well. Between 1 and 3 PM, the chi focuses on the Small Intestine and supplying energy to remove fluids and other nutrients from food as it progresses through the digestive tract. If your cat feels consistently uncomfortable during the Small Intestine time, it bears further investigation.

2. Listening and Smelling

The next phase relies on your senses of hearing and smelling. Listen to your cat's vocalization, respiration, heart, and abdominal sounds. Is there any wheezing sound or congested breathing? Is his heart pounding loudly? Any rumbling along his digestive tract? These can be indicators of imbalances in specific organ systems.

Raspy and congested breathing or wheezing would indicate a possible Lung imbalance. Heart pounding suggests a Heart or Pericardium imbalance. And, pronounced digestive tract sounds can indicate any of the zang-fu organs involved in digestion. Stomach, Spleen, Small Intestine, Large Intestine are the main organ systems responsible for taking in food and water, breaking them down into absorbable nutrients, and ridding the body of waste.

Strong smells tend to be associated with excess heat syndromes. When the weather is warm, we can smell the sweet fragrance of a flower. On cold, chilly days, the flower may still be in bloom, but we are apt not to smell it. Body secretions and excretions have some smell but should not be extremely smelly.

When your cat emits a strong odor, it usually means he's suffering from a heat condition. An example of a heat pattern or syndrome is an ear infection that usually has a distinct, strong odor.

Minimal or no odor suggests a cold or deficiency-type syndrome or pattern. For instance, when your cat's feces don't smell, this means he's not "cooking" his food well enough. Feces are supposed to smell. This indicates his Stomach and Spleen aren't processing and breaking down his food into absorbable nutrients, hence his stool doesn't smell like waste.

Foul and sour body odors usually indicate retention of food. Specific odors are associated with each of the zang organs and can be used to ascertain the nature and origin of the imbalance.

3. Questions / Inquiry

The next step in collecting information about your cat's condition is asking questions. It may seem strange to be asking yourself these questions if you are working with your own cat, but it's still a valuable process. Because you are familiar with your cat, you may miss important indicators. Asking good questions will clarify and expand your view.

With the current clinical signs in mind, start with general questions and progress to more specific ones to differentiate a particular pattern of disharmony.

Possible questions: How old is your cat? Has your cat been neglected, abused, abandoned, or injured at any time? Is he an indoor and/or outdoor cat? Does he have a friendly nature or is he aloof? Is he timid or fearful? Are there other cats or dogs in the family and how does he get along with them? Does he like cold weather or warm weather? In which season is he most active? What is his daily routine for eating, exercising, sleeping, and defecating/urinating? Does he eat raw, dry manufactured or canned food? Is he on medication? Has he had medical procedures in the past? Has he received inoculations lately? Is he fed supplements?

You could continue to ask many more questions, but this is a good start in knowing your cat's general daily existence. Now list any clinical signs of his current condition. Is your cat in pain or showing signs of weakness? Has he had any recent changes in behavior? Is he restless or lethargic? At what time of day is he restless or uncomfortable?

What picture is forming about your cat's lifestyle and how he's coping within his environment? You can ask more questions to understand his nature as well as his exposure to external factors and internal stressors related to his current condition. For instance, have you recently installed new carpet? Which household cleaners do you use? Do you use fertilizers on your lawn or garden? It's possible your cat may be reacting to toxic chemicals without your realizing it.

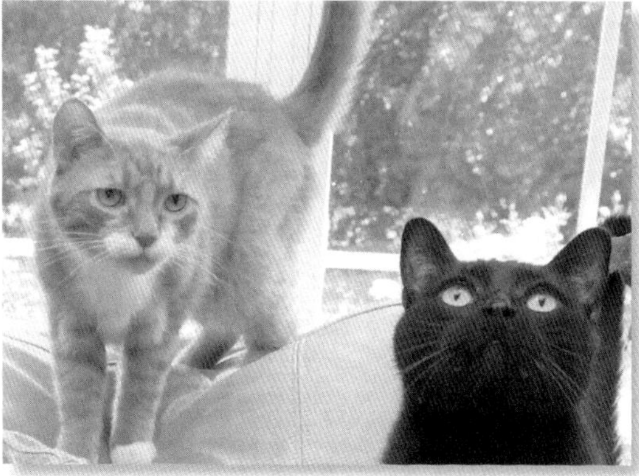

All of these inquiries are part of the puzzle for understanding your cat's condition. In Eastern medicine, we want to have as full a picture as possible because the acupoints selected for the session need to be specific for your cat.

If you suspect your cat has been exposed to toxic chemicals or his condition is deteriorating, have a veterinarian check him immediately. Also, if there's a sudden change in behavior, have your cat seen by a veterinarian. Remember, acupressure is a complementary therapy, not a substitute for veterinary care.

4. Physical Palpation

The last segment in assessing your cat's condition is extensive. All of the steps entail touching him as much as he will allow. Start with the general physical by going over his entire body gently but with intent. Don't force him to accept your touch if he's resistant. Simply try again later or on another day. Because you want this to be a good experience, there's no reason to force anything on your cat. In time, he will probably come to trust your healing intent and enjoy having you touch him all over. Cats have their own ideas about being touched, and we have to respect them.

Cats have their own ideas about being touched, and we have to respect them.

Feel for temperature. Are there differences in temperature? Is he hot or cold or just right? Do some of his muscles feel tight, atrophied, or well-toned? Can you feel any areas of tension, heat, or cold? Did your cat flinch when you touched a particular location? Is there any swelling, edema, a mass? Does his coat feel evenly smooth? Write down everything you feel and notice. Remember, all palpation should be reasonably gentle because you don't want to "spank the crying baby" and cause further pain or injury.

During this fourth phase of The Four Examinations, you're seeking more information about your cat's physical condition, adding to what you already learned during your observation, listening and smelling, and inquiry phases. You are looking for a distinguishing pattern telling you which, if any, of his organ systems is not balanced.

For instance, you've noticed that your 14-year-old cat isn't running to greet you at the door anymore when you come home. You smell his ears to check for infection and feel in and around them for any heat in the area or a pain reaction. There doesn't seem to be any heat or pain related to an infection, but given his age, it's not unusual for a cat to have a loss of hearing. Hearing is related to Kidney function. In this case, your cat, because of his age, is probably dealing with loss of hearing rooted in the diminishment of original Source chi. This distinguishing pattern points to a loss of Kidney chi.

Pulses

In TCM physical assessment, pulses are a major indicator of internal organ imbalance. Pulses on a cat are usually taken along the femoral artery located on the medial side of the hind leg. Although pulses are an important part of physical palpation in TCM, teaching them in an introductory book would not be appropriate because it takes years of practice to become proficient. Practitioners feel for a particular location of a pulse that corresponds to specific organ systems. They want to determine whether or not the pulses are superficial or deep, rapid or slow, strong or weak, wide or narrow, thick or wiry—plus many other qualities a pulse can indicate.

A highly detailed study, understanding pulses requires years of training. To simplify for introductory purposes, a rapid pulse usually indicates a heat syndrome while a slow pulse indicates a cold syndrome. In TCM, interpreting pulses is complex and goes beyond the scope of this book.

... rapid pulse usually indicates a heat syndrome while a slow pulse indicates a cold syndrome.

Association and Alarm Points

Two classifications of acupressure points are commonly used to assess the animal during the physical palpation segment of the Four Examinations. They are Association points and Alarm points. These assessment points narrow the focus one step further by directly touching and feeling the energetic activity of each zang-fu organ system.

The Association points, Back Transporting or Back *Shu* points, are located along the inner channel of the Bladder meridian. Each of the Association points is directly connected to the zang-fu organ for which it's named. The acupoints included in this category receive energy from the zang-fu organ and its related meridian. Because of this internal-external

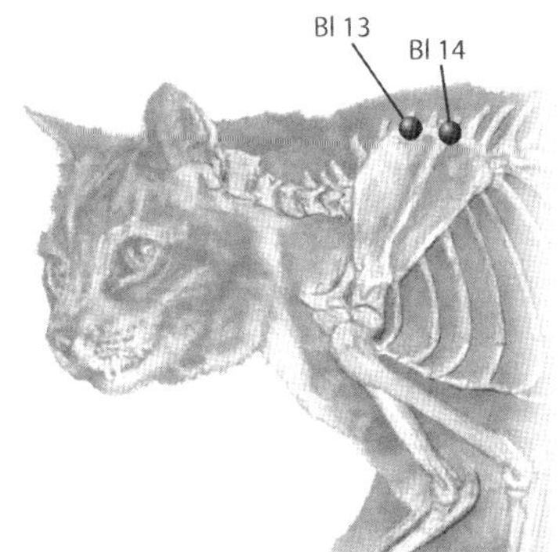

Bladder 13 – Lung Association Pt.
Bladder 14 – Pericardium Association Point

relationship with each of the organ systems, these points can communicate the condition of each organ system for assessment purposes.

For instance, by holding the soft tip of your thumb at a 45° to 90° angle to the cat's body on Bladder 13 (Bl 13), which is the Lung Association point, you can feel if the point is hot, cold, sinking, protruding, reactive, or normal. If Bl 13 feels cold and lifeless, there's most likely an imbalance in the Lung organ system (i.e., the lung organ itself and the meridian) of a cold nature.

Bladder 14 (Bl 14) is the Back-Shu point for the Pericardium, the sac surrounding the heart. When other indicators point to an imbalance in the Pericardium and possibly within the organ, you can check Bl 14 to detect if your cat is reactive or if you can feel any heat, coolness, softness, hardness, sinking – anything other than smooth and even. Information during the palpation phase of the Four Examinations provides one more indicator of an imbalance related to a particular organ system and its nature.

Alarm points, or Front-Mu points, further identify the depth and nature of an imbalance within a specific organ system. The Alarm points are found on the ventral (underside) or ventrolateral (lower-side) aspect of the cat. These acupoints are where chi of a zang-fu organ accumulates when the organ is suffering from an imbalance. Once the imbalance or disease has reached the zang-fu organs, the cat will most likely react to light thumb pressure on these points. Be careful to apply very light pressure when checking the Alarm points.

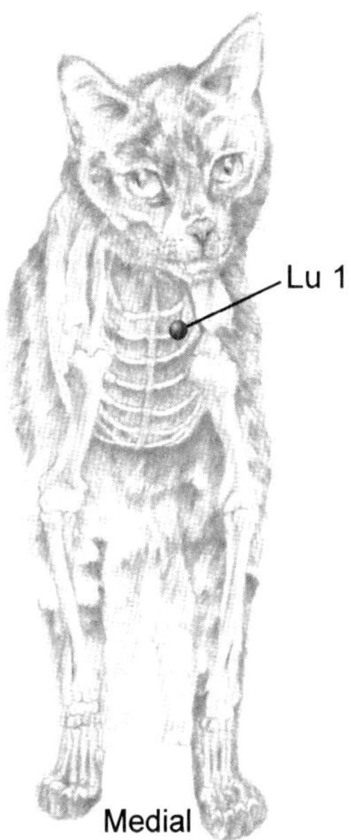

Lung 1 - Alarm Point

When the Association point for the Lung (Bladder 13) is reactive or indicates an imbalance, check Lung 1, the Alarm point for the

Lung, to find out if the imbalance has gone beyond the meridian level of the animal and is affecting the Lung organ. The Alarm points tell you if there's organ involvement in the imbalance.

Here's an example of how to work with Association and Alarm points. Your cat is urinating frequently. You first check to see if the Association points for the Kidney and Bladder, Bladder 23 and Bladder 28 respectively show any indication of heat or cold or feel different than the rest of her body. If you do feel something you will know she's experiencing an imbalance within the Bladder and/or Kidney organ and meridian. Now check the Kidney and Bladder Alarm points, Gall Bladder 25 and Conception Vessel 3 respectively to see if your cat reacts or the Alarm points feel different than the rest of her body. If she does react to one or both Alarm points, you will know there's organ involvement. If she does not react to either of these Alarm points, even though you felt something on the Association points, then the issue is superficial and at the meridian level of her body. When the imbalance is at the meridian level you can use specific acupoints to bring it back into balance.

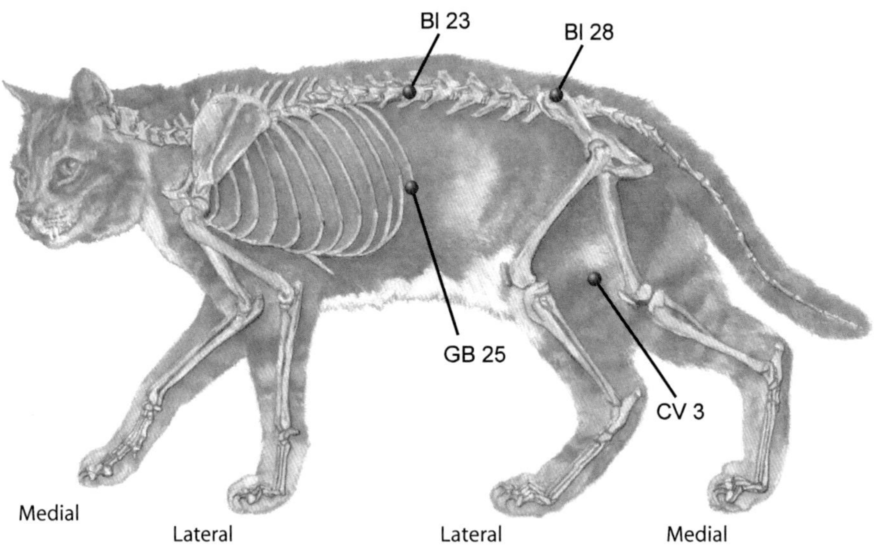

Acupoints to use when assessing a Urinary Issues

Bladder 23 and **Bladder 28** – Association Points for Kidney and Bladder respectively
Gall Bladder 25 and **Conception Vessel 3** – Alarm Points for Kidney and Bladder respectively

To review, the Association points indicate when the zang-fu organ system is experiencing an imbalance. By checking the Alarm points, you will learn if the imbalance is easily dealt with on a meridian level or if the imbalance lies deeper in your cat's body and is affecting the internal organ(s). Remember this doesn't mean there's any form of organ disease, it simply means that there's an imbalance and the organ is not functioning optimally.

Both the Association and Alarm points provide invaluable information for assessing a cat's condition because they narrow the imbalance to particular organ systems and provide indicators regarding the nature of the imbalance. These two classifications of acupoints are part of the Opening Sequence of the Feline Acupressure Session Protocol discussed in Chapter 7.

Using The Four Examinations to assess your cat is extremely important in figuring out how to help him feel his best. When you are a beginner, it may seem to take a long time to move through each of the four phases. However, with practice plus the more you know about the functions of the zang-fu organs, the more proficient and easy the assessment process will become.

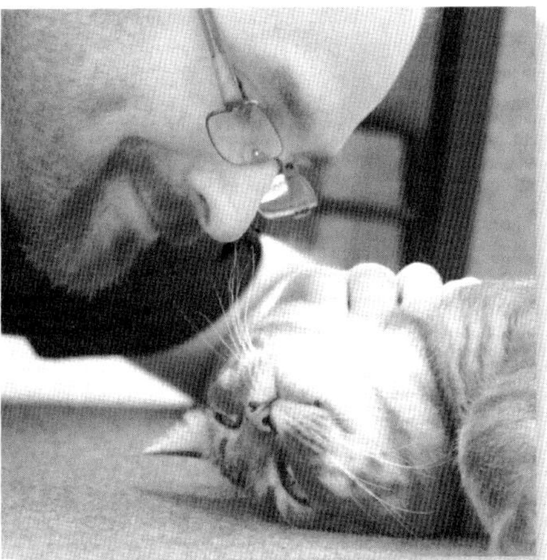

"The great thing about cats is their endless variety. One can pick a cat to fit almost any kind of décor, income, personality, mood. But under the fur, there still lies, essentially unchanged, one of the world's free souls."

— Eric Gurney

Traditional Chinese Medicine List of Concepts

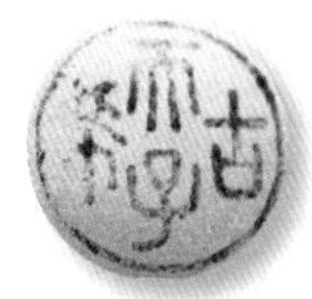

Law of Integrity

The body is a whole:
What is occurring internally manifests externally

Five Stems of Chinese Medicine

- Acupuncture / Acupressure
- Tui Na (Meridian Massage)
- Diet
- Chi Gong (Exercise Technique)
- Herbs

Functions of Chi

Promotes	Controls
Warms	Activates
Defends	Nourishes

Yin-Yang Theory

- Opposites
- Interdependent
- Mutually consuming
- Transform into each other
- Pattern of Disharmony –
  - Excess –
    - Yang: Sedate Yang
    - Yin: Sedate Yin
  - Deficiency –
    - Yang: Tonify Yang
    - Yin: Tonify Yin

Zang – Fu & Meridian Theory

- 12 Major Organs / Meridians –
  - Lung / Large Intestine
  - Stomach / Spleen
  - Heart / Small Intestine
  - Bladder / Kidney
  - Pericardium / Triple Heater
  - Gall Bladder / Liver
  - Two Extraordinary Vessels –
    - Conception Vessel
    - Governing Vessel

Five-Element Theory

Wood	Earth	Water
Fire	Metal	

The Four Examinations

- Observation
- Listening / Smelling
- Questions / Inquiry
- Physical Palpation
  - Association points
  - Alarm points

Vital Substances

- Chi
- Blood
- Body Fluids

Eight Principles

- Exterior – Interior
- Hot – Cold
- Excess – Deficiency
- Yin – Yang

Chapter Seven

Feline Acupressure Session Protocol

The acupressure session starts when you and your cat connect. With your cat relaxed and purring next to you on the couch, it's a good time to begin a session. If your cat is active and wants to play, enjoy playtime and wait until he is ready for a rest.

Remember, an acupressure session is a dynamic, energetic interaction between two equal partners – you and your cat. You bring a clear intention to enhance the cat's health and well-being to your role.

... an acupressure session is a dynamic, energetic interaction between two equal partners – you and your cat.

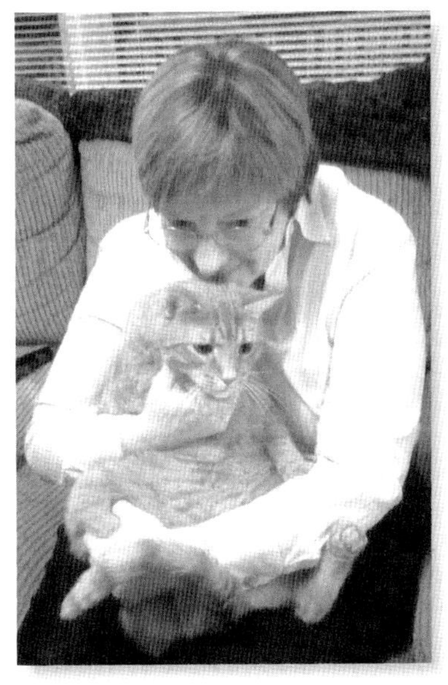

For you to fulfill your role, you must be consciously present. Let all of life's pressures and concerns fall away. Take six to eight deep, even breaths and allow yourself to exhale down to the bottom of your breath. As you exhale, follow the vibration of your breath across the room and away from you. Feel yourself release any tension in your body. If thoughts of your grocery list arise, just breathe them away. Then take your next three breaths, focus on your heart opening to your highest intent. Your job is to be there for your cat at this moment.

Because cats are sensitive, they know when we are attempting to connect with them, even when they choose to ignore us.

It may take a few sessions to become comfortable with each other because intentional touch is different from simple petting and showing affection. Your cat may take some time to trust your therapeutic intention. After all, cats don't like to be restrained. It would be counterproductive to have a frantic cat scrambling to get away. Your cat needs to be able to connect with his internal energy during the session for the acupressure to be most effective.

Once your cat is accustomed to participating in an acupressure session, he will consider it a treat! Actually, many cats become rather demanding of their right to an acupressure session. In time, many cats help guide their guardians through a session because they know what they need. So be alert to the directions your cat is giving you. Allowing him to communicate his needs is a significant part of sharing this experience.

Remember, the key to an effective session is the intimate interaction between you and your cat.

Feline Acupressure Session Protocol

There are three major segments of a comprehensive acupressure session that happen before, during, and after the session. The "before" portion is the Pre-Session segment. That's when you will (1) select a location, (2) prepare yourself, (3) introduce yourself to the cat and gain permission, and (4) begin the assessment process.

Selecting a Location – Find a comfortable location where there are few distractions. Because cats like to be in their own territory, they generally are more relaxed at home. You want your cat to feel safe so you can both focus on the exchange of

Acupressure Session

Pre-Session

Selecting a location

Preparing yourself

Introducing yourself and gaining permission

Assessment process - Four Examinations

Session Phases

Opening

Point work

Closing

Post-Session

Observation

energy that occurs during the session. Pay attention. If the chi and blood supply to your legs are cut off by the way you're sitting, it will detract from your session. Your free flow of blood and chi is important for your cat to gain benefit from the session.

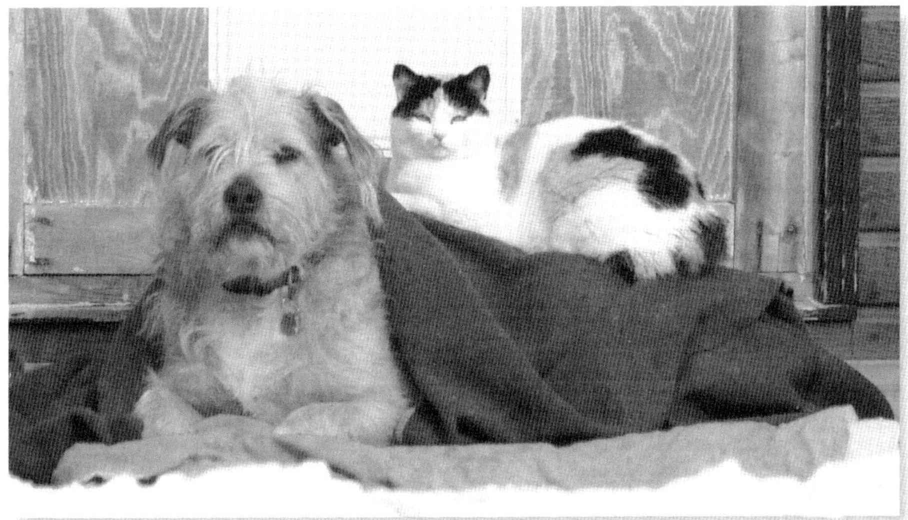

If other animals in the home are around, they usually want to be close by and even snuggle in while the session is in progress. These animals could be receiving the energetic shifts even though you're not touching them directly. As long as you and your cat feel at ease and the other animals aren't distracting, everyone can enjoy the session together.

Allow your cat to find his own position on the bed, the couch, or your lap. The less you fuss with your cat, the more open he will be to the bodywork. You can encourage your cat to stay with you but don't restrain him. If he adamantly resists, try to settle into a session later or on another day. There's no reason to force an acupressure session.

Preparing Yourself – Breathing helps you relax and become present. As mentioned in the beginning of this chapter, inhale deeply and exhale to the bottom of your breath six to eight times. As you exhale, follow the vibration of your breath as it travels away from you. Let your mind go blank for a few moments and feel your worries and the demands of the day drift far away.

Formulating your healing intention for the session is essential to a successful outcome. Take a few minutes to focus on your cat and think about how you want him to feel his best physically and emotionally. The quality of the session is greatly enhanced by your healing intent. Do you want your cat to heal from a specific illness or injury? Are you most interested in his remaining balanced and healthy? Your intention provides the impetus for the entire acupressure session.

Introducing Yourself and Gaining Permission – Because cats are sensitive, living, sentient beings, they appreciate it when you introduce yourself before touching them. You can introduce yourself silently or verbally, or simply by picturing the process in your mind. It would be good to let your cat know you are going to enjoy sharing healing moments with him.

Look for signals that tell you your cat is giving you permission to touch him. These signals can take a variety of forms such as turning toward you, leaning into you, softening his eyes, lying down, or communicating energetically. When your cat gives no response, try moving to another location and ask for permission again. If, after three attempts to work with him and he's still unresponsive, honor his choice not to have an acupressure session at that time. Ask again some other time.

Beginning the Assessment Process – Humans are given to first impressions. The moment you see your cat, you've begun the assessment process even though you are not assessing the animal formally during that instant. You can tell a lot about an animal within a second or two including: the brightness of his eyes, his general conformation, and the attitude he presents.

The assessment process begins with a broad, general view and increasingly narrows the focus to arrive at a current pattern of disharmony. The Four Examinations, as discussed in Chapter Six, may seem like a crude assessment tool given modern technology. When you study eastern pathology and finely tune your senses, the Four Examinations offer you a refined method of assessing your cat's health. Modern technology definitely has its place in the assessment process. Still, Chinese medicine practitioners are known to detect health issues that are subclinical by using their finely honed senses and extensive knowledge of zang-fu patterns.

The Pre-Session assessment process is your initial impression of your cat's condition. Are his eyes bright? Is he moving well? Does his coat feel smooth and appear healthy? In this process, you're looking for your cat's general appearance, conformation, and sense of vitality.

Phases of the Acupressure Session

Opening Phase

In Chinese medicine, one phase blends into another; there are few hard lines of division from one phase of the acupressure protocol to the next. The acupressure session begins with the fourth phase of the Four Examinations, the Physical Palpation segment. The reason to include the physical in the Opening Phase of the acupressure session is that when you touch your cat, you have begun balancing chi and blood. Simply by virtue of your touch, the cat's energetic balance starts to shift.

"Just by virtue of your touch, the cat's energetic balance is starting to shift."

Performing a physical during the Opening Phase marks the moment you narrow your focus and begin to identify, or discern, specific issues related to the indicators your cat is exhibiting.

For the general physical, gently touch your cat all over his body. You are feeling for swelling, hard lumps, edema, or any unusual variations in his coat as well as muscle tone and temperature balance. Note anything that is not within the norm for your cat.

Bladder Meridian

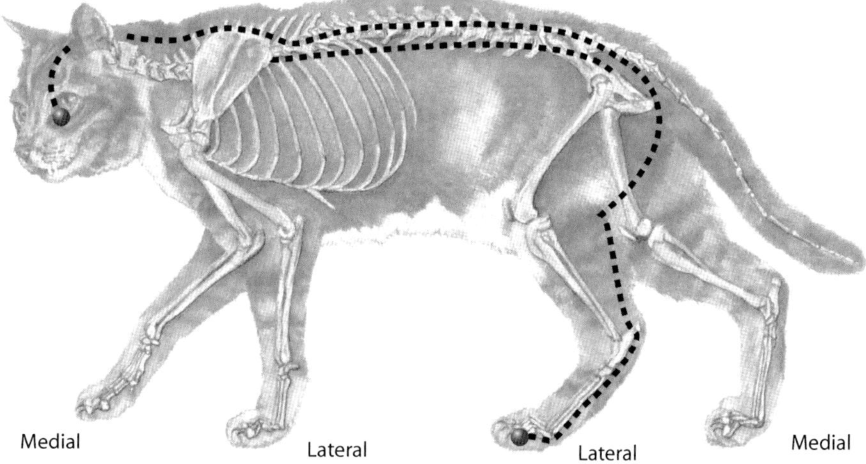

The Opening is performed on the Bladder meridian.

The next step entails using the thenar prominence, which is the soft portion of your palm before your thumb on the heel of your hand. With minimal pressure, trace the Bladder meridian located on the dorsal aspect, or back, of the cat approximately one inch away from the spine. (See Bladder meridian chart on preceding page.)

Although the Bladder meridian begins at the inner corner, or inner canthus, of the cat's eye, start tracing the meridian on the cat's neck. Most cats prefer this starting point. Glide the heel of your hand slowly and evenly along the Bladder meridian, feeling for hot or cold areas and hard or soft spots. Rest your other hand comfortably somewhere on the cat's body. The resting hand serves as an anchor that connects you with your cat.

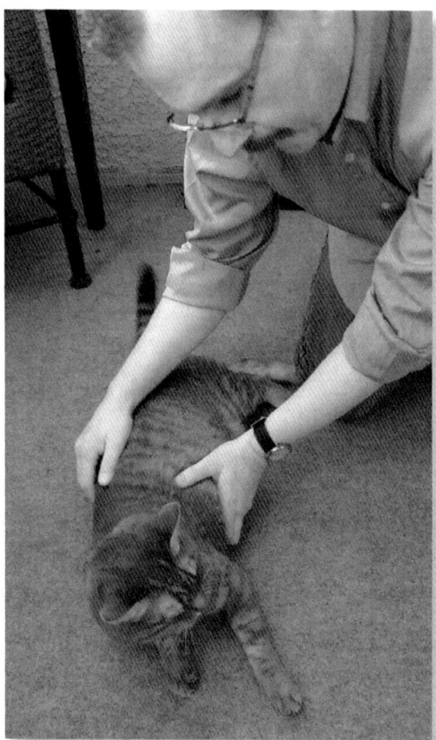
Tracing the Bladder meridian

Continue tracing the Bladder meridian down the cat's back toward the tail, then down the hind leg to the outside, or lateral aspect, of the cat's fifth digit. Repeat this procedure, starting on the neck and tracing the meridian three times on each side of the cat.

By performing the Opening Phase, you communicate that you and your cat are engaging in something other than a petting session; you're telling him you're about to begin intentional touch.

While performing the Opening by tracing the Bladder meridian, pay attention to the temperature of each section on the cat's back. The temperature can offer a glimpse at what could be occurring internally. For instance, an older cat may feel cool in the loin area, indicating a possible imbalance related to the Kidney meridian. This doesn't mean something alarming such as kidney disease. Rather, it could simply be an imbalance you can attend to easily and manage by selecting acupoints that enhance Kidney chi.

When you've completed tracing the Bladder meridian three times on each side of the cat during the Opening, note any temperature changes, sensitivities, lumps, indents, protrusions, soft or hard areas. At this moment during the Opening procedure, write down any of these you can feel and note where it is located. Doing this prepares you for the next step that will yield more definitive information.

The Association points (also called Back Shu points) are a classification of acupoints that share the attribute of being internally connected with the zang-fu organ for which they're named. These points are used during the Opening because they can indicate how the organ system is functioning. If the Association point feels cold, there may be other indicators pointing to an imbalance within the related meridian or the organ itself. For example, Bladder 23 (Bl 23) is the Kidney Association point. When this point feels cool, it may indicate an imbalance along the Kidney meridian.

Additionally, the Association point on one side of the cat may not feel the same on the opposite side. Think of these points as providing one more piece of information to add to other indicators gathered during the Four Examinations.

It is easy to distinguish bone from muscle on a strong, lean cat, though the length and density of his fur may be an issue when finding an acupoint. On a more full-figured cat, locating an acupoint may prove tricky. Just take your time locating the acupoints.

For their small size, a healthy cat is remarkable strong. Just try to do something your cat doesn't want you to do and you will find out how strong he is.

The Association point for the Pericardium (the sac surrounding and protecting the Heart located in the thoracic region of the cat's body) is Bladder 14 (Bl 14). Say your cat reacts when you touch that point with the soft tip of your thumb. You recognize that Bl 14 feels warmer than the other surrounding area. You've also noticed that the cat seems apprehensive and particularly wary of strangers in general. His body language and look in his eyes tell you he is defensive. These behaviors, plus the warm sensation of Bl 14, indicate the cat is having trust issues. As noted earlier, trust is related to the functioning of the Pericardium.

Using the soft tip of your thumb at a 45-to-90° angle to the surface of the cat's back, gently feel each one of the 12 Association points starting with Bladder 13, the Association point for the Lung. Note any temperature and texture differences. It's important to be conscious of any sensitivity to a specific point the cat may have.

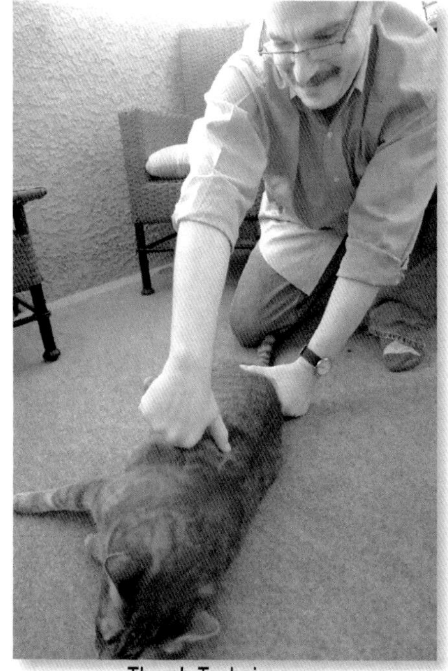
Thumb Technique on Association point

Remember, encourage but don't force your cat to participate in an acupressure session. For their small size, a healthy cat is quite strong.

At first, when you're learning, this process seems to take a long time and requires a lot of concentration. True, it does at first. But once you become familiar with the assessment process, it will become second nature and flow becomes seamless.

It is common to feel awkward when learning new skills plus it takes time to train your hands and trust what you feel. The only way to get beyond this stage is constant practice. People become proficient by practicing with their own cats, their brothers' cats, their neighbors' cats, shelter cats, and so on. That's the best way to learn.

After checking each of the Association points and noting anything significant, you can move on to checking the Alarm points, also called Front Mu points, to discern if the imbalance is superficial—that is, only within the meridian—or if it's deeper in the body and affecting the organ. Because meridians are just beneath the surface of the skin, they're considered relatively superficial. The Association points can reveal imbalances within the organ system. The Alarm points provide the next piece of information: how deeply has the imbalance penetrated into the body and has it affected the organ itself?

There are 12 Alarm points that correlate with the 12 Major Meridians. The Alarm points are located on the ventral aspect, or underside, of the cat's trunk. These Alarm points signify where the chi of a particular organ gathers when an organ is imbalanced.

Another example of how to use the Association and Alarm points is while working with a cat with a history of urinary problems, the practitioner checks Bladder 23 and 28 (the Association points for Kidney and Bladder respectively) and the cat moves away. This means the cat is likely indicating these points are uncomfortable. As a result, the practitioner becomes aware that this cat may have an imbalance related to the Kidney and Bladder meridians.

The next step is to check the Kidney and Bladder Alarm points to see if the cat reacts to them. The Alarm point for the Kidney is Gall Bladder 25 (GB 25) and the Alarm point for the Bladder is Conception Vessel (CV 3). When the cat exhibits sensitivity upon palpating Alarm points, a disruption in organ function is probable. If the cat doesn't react to working the Alarm point, then the imbalance is most likely on the superficial meridian level of the cat's body and hasn't penetrated more deeply.

We tend to assess the Alarm points only when something is indicated by the corresponding Association point or when other indicators lead to a pattern of disharmony related to an organ. This is part of understanding the nature of the imbalance and leads directly to the next phase of the acupressure protocol, the acupoint selection for the Point Work.

Here's another example of performing an assessment to determine the pattern of disharmony. Let's say Bink, a large, elderly, neutered male, seems to be straining when he goes to the litter box. He has not defecated in about two days. In addition, his lower abdomen is bloated and he isn't grooming himself well. When performing the physical the Large Intestine Association point, you noted Bladder 25 (Bl 25) was quite warm. In addition, Bink squirmed away when Stomach 25, the Alarm point for the Large Intestine, was palpated. These reactions indicate that Bink may be experiencing a Large Intestine pattern of disharmony.

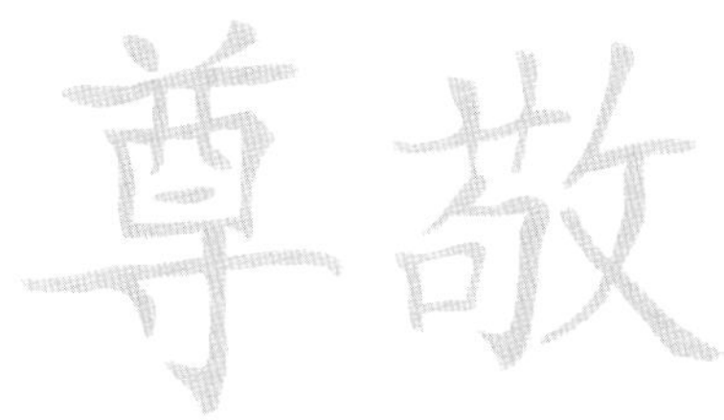

Association Points

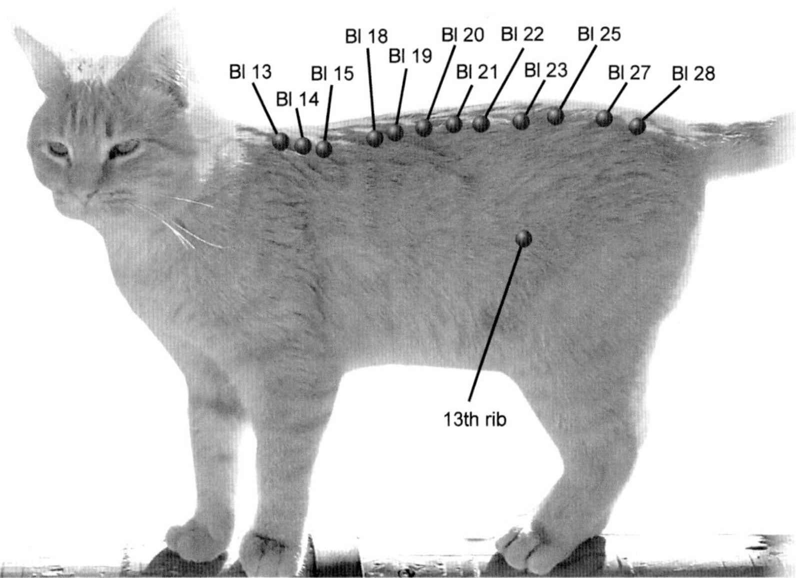

Point	Meridian – Location
Bl 13	Lung –1.5 cun lateral to back edge dorsal spinous process of 3rd thoracic vertebra.
Bl 14	Pericardium – 1.5 cun lateral to back edge of dorsal spinous process of 4th thoracic vertebra.
Bl 15	Heart –1.5 cun lateral to back edge of dorsal spinous process of 5th thoracic vertebra.
Bl 18	Liver – 1.5 cun lateral to back edge of dorsal spinous process of 10th thoracic vertebra.
Bl 19	Gall Bladder – 1.5 cun lateral to back edge of dorsal spinous process of 11th thoracic vertebra.
Bl 20	Spleen – 1.5 cun lateral to back edge of dorsal spinous process of 12th thoracic vertebra.
Bl 21	Stomach – 1.5 cun lateral to caudal border of dorsal spinous process of 13th thoracic vertebra.
Bl 22	Triple Heater – 1.5 cun lateral to caudal border of dorsal spinous process of 1st lumbar vertebra.
Bl 23	Kidney – 1.5 cun lateral to back edge of dorsal spinous process of 2nd lumbar vertebra.
Bl 25	Large Intestine – 1.5 cun lateral to caudal border of dorsal spinous process of 5th lumbar vertebra.
Bl 27	Small Intestine – 1.5 cun lateral to caudal border of dorsal spinous process of 7th lumbar vertebra.
Bl 28	Bladder – Located lateral to 2nd foramen, in depression between sacrum and medial border of dorsal iliac spine.

Alarm Points

Alarm points can be used in both assessment and for point work.

Meridian	Alarm Point
Lung	Lu 1
Large Intestine	St 25
Stomach	CV 12
Spleen	Liv 13
Heart	CV 14
Small Intestine	CV 4
Bladder	CV 3
Kidney	GB 25
Pericardium	CV 17
Triple Heater	CV 5
Gall Bladder	GB 24
Liver	Liv 14

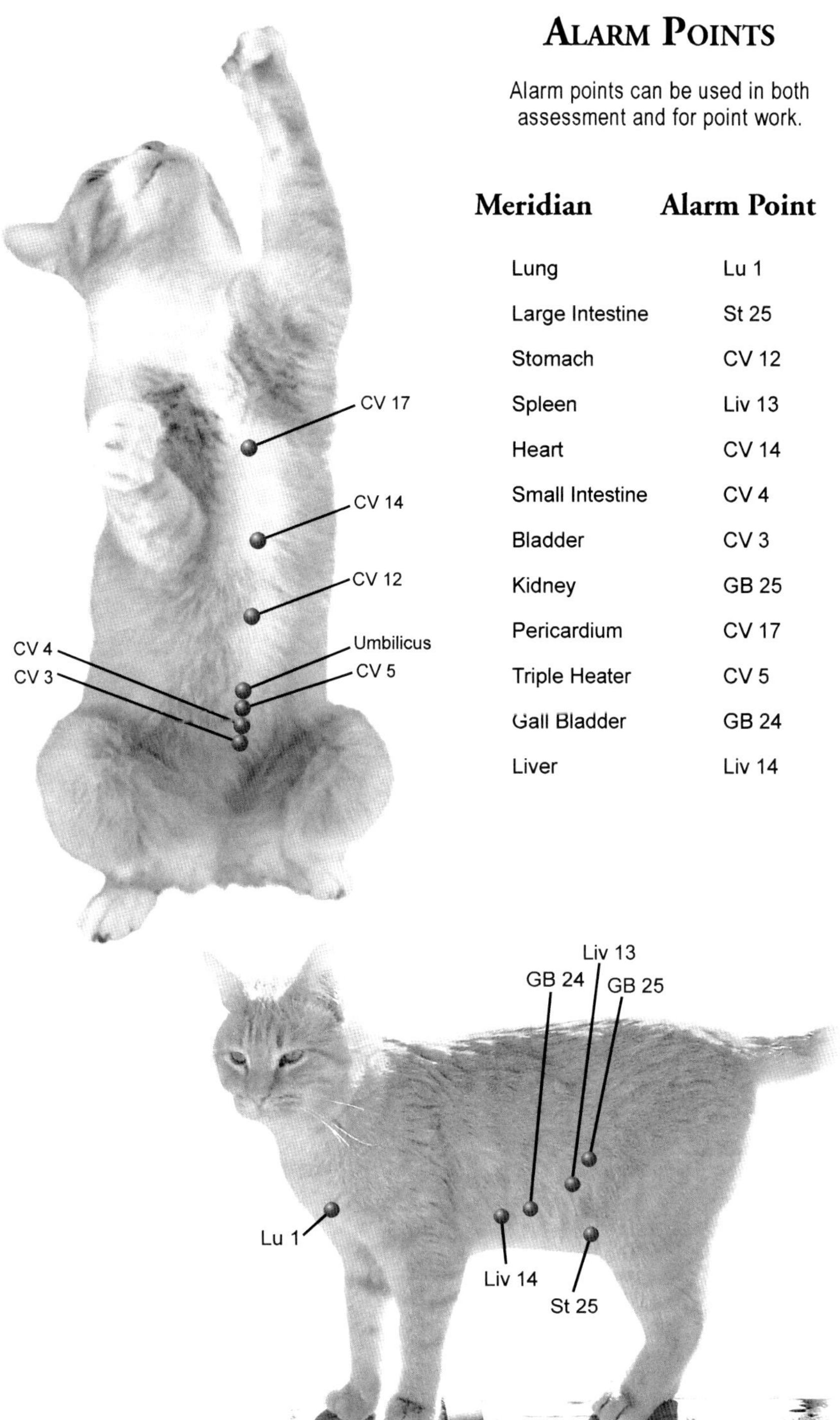

Again, as you feel each Association point going down the Bladder meridian, note any temperature or texture changes. If you feel any irregularity at an Association point, check the corresponding Alarm point.

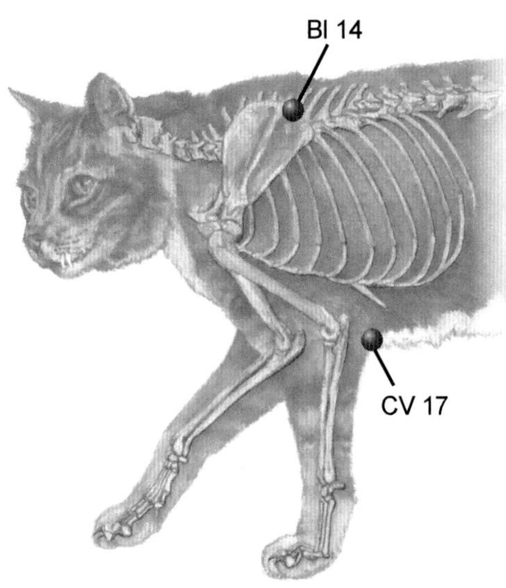

Bladder 14 and **Conception Vessel 17**

If Bladder 14 (Bl 14), the Association point for the Pericardium, feels warm, then gently check the Alarm point for the Pericardium, Conception Vessel 17 (CV 17) to see if the cat is reactive on that acupoint. If the cat seems to be uncomfortable when you touch CV 17, know that he's experiencing an imbalance of the Pericardium.

During the physical palpation segment, your cat may not give you any response or feedback. Cats like to keep secrets and they can be stoic about their hurts, at this point, rely on the other assessment information you have collected while going through the Four Examinations. Your observations provide valid information on which to base your assessment.

After completing the physical palpation section of the Four Examinations, including the Association and Alarm points, review all the information you have collected about your cat. Then use your knowledge of the functions of the zang-fu organ systems to arrive at which organ system is not balanced.

One more example - Tuffy has not been eating as much as usual. She seems tired all the time although she appears to be most uncomfortable in the morning before you leave for work at 8AM. You check her Association points for Spleen and Stomach, Bladder 20 and 21 (Bl 20 and 21), the Association points for the Spleen and Stomach respectively, and they feel a bit cool. Then you check the Spleen and Stomach Alarm points, Liver 13 (Liv 13) and Conception Vessel 12 (CV 12) respectively and she does not react; both Alarm points feel normal. Given these indicators, you can surmise that Tuffy is likely experiencing a digestion problem that is relatively superficial and can be resolved on the meridian level since it has not gone deeper into her body. If she had reacted to the Alarm points we could guess that Tuffy's digestive condition had affected her internal organs. Luckily, this Spleen-Stomach imbalance or pattern of disharmony can be quickly resolved by balancing the Spleen and Stomach meridians.

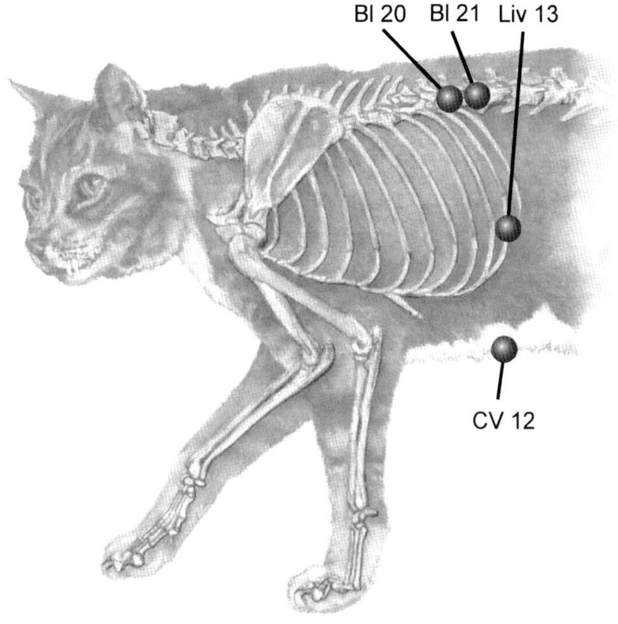

Bladder 20 and **Bladder 21** – Association Points for Spleen and Stomach respectively; **Liver 13** and **Conception Vessel 12** – Alarm Points for Spleen and Stomach respectively

Zang-Fu Theory, the core of eastern pathology, directs you toward the specific organ system(s) that require balancing. (Review Chapter Six for a detailed explanation of the assessment process.) Because this is a hands-on activity, at this point in your learning, it would be good to receive hands-on training. Written words alone cannot take the place of seeing, feeling, and doing the procedures with the guidance of a knowledgeable instructor. This book serves as a general guide.

Point Selection Process

Assessment

- **Four Examinations**
  - **Observation**
  - **Listening / Smelling**
  - **Inquiry / Questions**
  - **Physical palpation**
    - **General physical**
    - **Association points**
    - **Alarm points**

Assessment Outcome

- **Current condition**
- **Identify meridian(s) / Organ system involvement**

Point Selection

- **Association point(s)**
- **Source point(s)**

Point Work

Selecting acupoints for the Point Work requires sufficient knowledge of Zang-Fu Theory and acupoint energetics and functions to make appropriate point selection. The goal is to pick points that are most effective in resolving the presenting health or behavioral issue.

An incredible number of point selection techniques have evolved over the centuries. In fact, entire books have been written describing a single point selection technique. Some are extremely complex while others are quite simple.

To introduce you to acupoint selection, it's best to start with a simple and direct method of selecting acupoints.

The Association points used during the assessment portion of the Opening are powerful acupoints because they're internally and externally connected to an organ. Association points can be of great benefit during the acupressure session as well as the assessment. These acupoints benefit chronic conditions such as arthritis. Bladder 23, the Kidney Association point, is commonly used for arthritic conditions because the Kidney function is related to bone.

Another example is the selection of Bladder 18 (Bl 18), the Liver Association point. When a Persian presents with continuous lacrimation (tearing of the eyes), you can use Bl 18, (the sense organ of the Liver is the eyes) to help resolve the eyes tearing excessively.

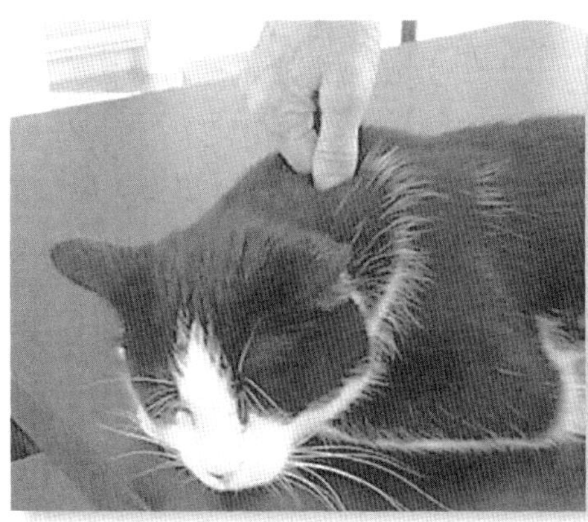

Thumb Technique: The meridians and acupoints are just beneath the surface of the skin, you won't need to press heavily or deeply.

Combining Association points with another category of points called Source, or *Yuan*, points creates a simple yet powerful selection of acupoints for the Point Work segment of the acupressure session.

Each of the 12 Major Meridians has it own Source point. Source chi is Original Essence chi with which the animal arrives on earth and inherits from its parents.

Source Points

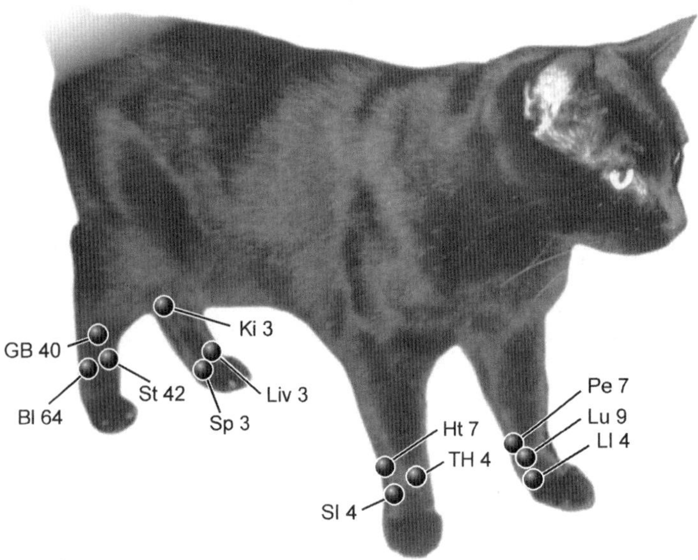

Point	Location
Lu 9	Located on the medial aspect of the radiocarpal joint, just cranial to the radial artery, at the level of Ht 7. Source point for Lung.
LI 4	Between 1st (dewclaw) and 2nd metacarpal bones, on medial side of 2nd metacarpal. Source point for Large Intestine.
St 42	Dorsal aspect of the tarsal joint, at the junction of the 3rd and 4th tarsal bones and the base of the 3rd and 4th metatarsal bones. Source point for Stomach.
Sp 3	Located on the mid-point of the medial aspect of the 2nd metatarsal bone. Source point for Spleen.
Ht 7	At the transverse crease of the carpal joint, in a depression lateral to the flexor carpi ulnaris. Opposite to Pe 7. Source point for Heart.
SI 4	On the ulnar border in a depression at the base of the 5th metacarpal bone. Source point for Small Intestine.
Bl 64	Located on the lateral aspect of the hind leg, in a depression below and behind the tuberosity of the 5th metatarsal bone. Source point for Bladder.
Ki 3	In the depression between the medial malleolus of the tibia and the calcaneal tendon. Opposite Bl 60. Source point for Kidney.
Pe 7	Caudal to tendon of the flexor carpi radialis and directly above the carpal bone. Source point for Pericardium.
TH 4	On the lateral side of the forelimb, at the radiocarpal joint, cranial to the tendon of the common digital extensor. Source point for Triple Heater.
GB 40	Lateral aspect of hind limb, on either side of the lateral malleolus of the fibula. Source point for Gall Bladder.
Liv 3	Between 2nd and 3rd metatarsal bones at junction of metatarsophalangeal joint. Source point for Liver.

If the queen is a black British Shorthair and the Tom is a black British Shorthair, most of the offspring will likely be black British Shorthairs. The kittens will arrive on earth with British shorthair Source chi. Because the parents are British shorthair cats, the kittens' Essence chi, or Source chi, will be the same; they will grow up to look like their parents.

When using Source points, you're working with the essence and fundamental chi of your cat.

Another important energetic characteristic of Source points is that they, when palpated, do what's necessary to balance the meridian. Source points respond to what the body requires at the time so the practitioner doesn't need to be concerned whether the condition is excess or deficient in nature. This attribute is highly significant, especially when you're first learning acupressure.

Knowing the functions of the organ systems is necessary for you to choose acupoints that will benefit your cat.

To select the appropriate Source point and Association point for a specific issue, refer to your assessment. A simple approach to point selection is based on Zang-Fu Theory. Knowing the functions of the organ systems is necessary for you to choose acupoints that will benefit your cat. For instance, when a cat is recuperating from oral surgery, select the Association and Source points related to the Spleen, Bladder 21, and Spleen 3 respectively because the Spleen is responsible for the health of the mouth.

By selecting Bladder 20 and Spleen 3 for your Point Work during the acupressure session, you will be working with four acupoints because acupoints are bilateral. It's recommended you perform Point Work on both sides of your cat.

The Point selection for a cat experiencing a loss of hearing would be the Kidney Association point, Bladder 23 (Bl 23), and the Source point on the Kidney meridian, Kidney 3 (Ki 3). The ears are the sense organ related to Kidney, which includes both the health of the ear and the acuity of hearing. Using these points bilaterally for the Point Work phase of the acupressure session provides the cat with therapeutic benefit for a hearing issue.

Acupoint Selection

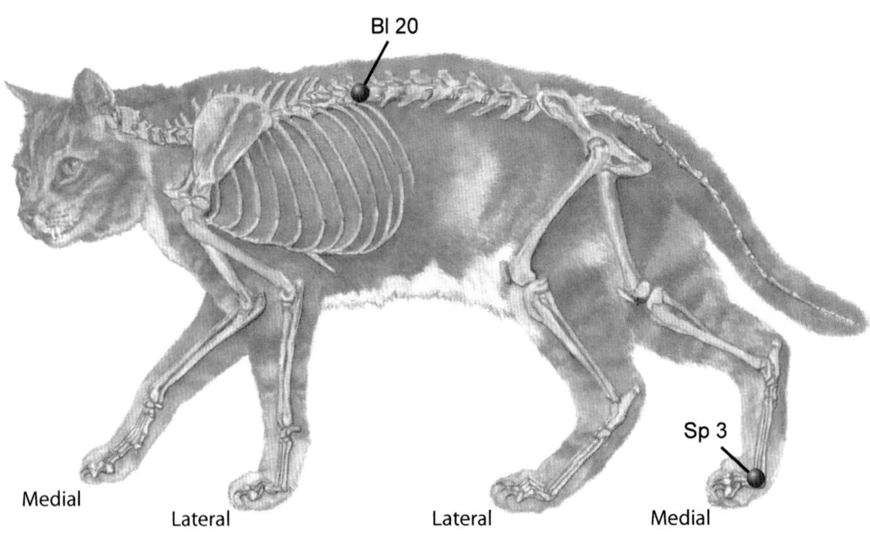

Association and Source points for mouth health:
Bladder 20 and **Spleen 3**

Bladder 13 (Bl 13), the Association point for the Lung, and Lung 9 (Lu 9), the Source point on the Lung meridian, combine to create the Point Work for a cat with respiratory issues. The Lung is responsible for all respiratory functions. These two acupoints (bilaterally) support the health of the Lung.

Point Work Techniques

It takes practice to educate your hands. That means tuning in and focusing on the sensations your hands and fingers are experiencing during the initial general physical (the Opening), during Point Work, and during the last segment of the acupressure session (the Closing). It takes considerable effort to become conscious of temperature changes and shifts in texture. Most acupressure practitioners reach the point of actually feeling chi move under their fingers, telling them a blockage or stagnation has released and chi is able to flow again.

Two Point Work techniques are the thumb technique and the two-finger technique.

Thumb Technique

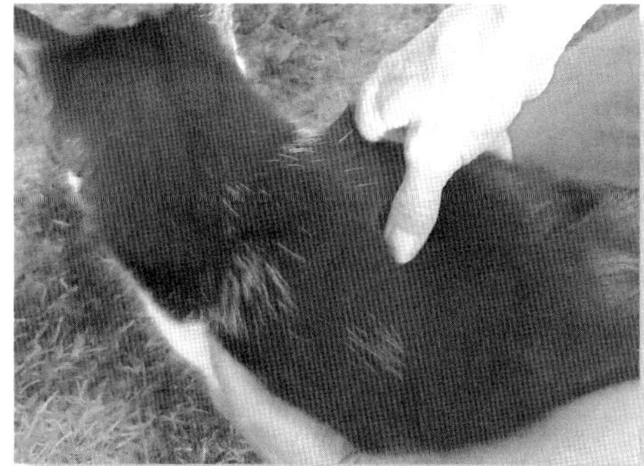
Thumb Technique

The thumb technique is used most frequently. It entails using the soft, fleshy portion of the tip of your thumb at a 45-to-90° angle to the cat's body. This technique is best for acupoints located on the cat's head, neck, and trunk.

Two-Finger Technique

Take your middle finger and place it on top the nail of your pointer finger to form a little tent. This is the two-finger technique. The point work is done with the soft tip of the pointer finger at a 45-to-90° angle from the cat's body. The two-finger technique is used along the cat's legs.

Point work technique is best described by following the concept projected in "Muddy Water," which follows.

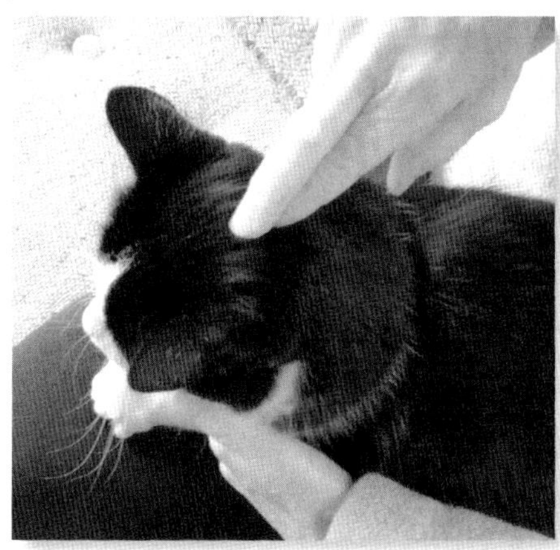
Two Finger Technique

The length of time you stay on an acupoint can vary. As a beginner, keep your thumb on an acupoint for a very slow count from 1 to 30 while feeling for any changes in the point and observing your cat. If he indicates discomfort with any pressure you're applying, please move on to the next point or discontinue the session. There's no reason for your cat to be uncomfortable during an acupressure session.

As your fingers become more educated, you will feel the flow of chi beneath the skin. There are different ways an acupoint can feel and, as you're "working" it, you may feel a shift in the energy. Sometimes it's as simple as feeling a cool point warming or a warm point cooling or a hard texture softening. Once the acupoint has shifted, it's time to move on.

Muddy Water
...the concept of Point Work Technique

The smooth-surfaced pond is clear and quiet, not even the smallest, softest ripple sullies the water.

If you were to plunge your hand into the pond and forcefully poke into the silt-layered bottom, spirals of tiny particles would rush up into the currents of water your hand created, disturbing the pool and obscuring your view and sense of what is beneath. By creating muddy water you would lose the ability to feel and know what really lays below that needs your attention.

But, when you gently cut the surface of this motionless pond and gently glide down to the bottom, the silt layers are revealed. You can feel and see what is there without creating a blinding torrent of silt and mud.

Kind, light touch on the first layer of silt bottom lets you know if there is pain. Come up a bit away to allow the slight drifting silt to settle back.

The first layer will give way to the second – rest the tip of your thumb momentarily on that place, what do you feel?

Is there a sense of energy in that place?
Is it dull, empty, cool, depressed?
Or, is it hot, protruding, angry?

It could be calm, mild, and smooth to the touch.

Come away from the point ever so slightly for a second, then return and gently be admitted to the third layer of silt, be content to stay there, not pressing, just hold that space.

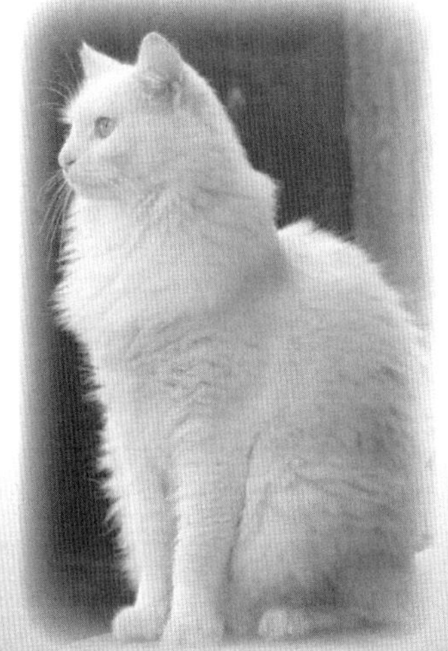

Energy has its own pace, we are here to encourage, not force, not rush.

Hold that point with healing intention and wait for any resistance barrier to give way, stay the course, the resistance will pass and you will be meeting the need for energy to break free and flow harmoniously.

While you're holding an acupoint, the cat may give signs that energy is moving in his body. These signs are called "releases" due to the stimulation of acupoints. These releases are the cat's reaction to the chi moving again as well as his body assisting in promoting the flow of chi. Releases include yawning, stretching, shaking, licking, rolling over, passing air, and sometimes even sleeping!

When you see and feel your cat releasing, stop holding the point and allow the natural process to run its course. Then go on to the next acupoint or, if the cat indicates he's done with the session, go ahead and perform the Closing described next.

Closing

The last phase of the acupressure session is the Closing. It's reconnecting the energy of the cat's body and tidying up any loose ends. Your intention is to have a definite end to the session and leave the cat with a complete gift of acupressure.

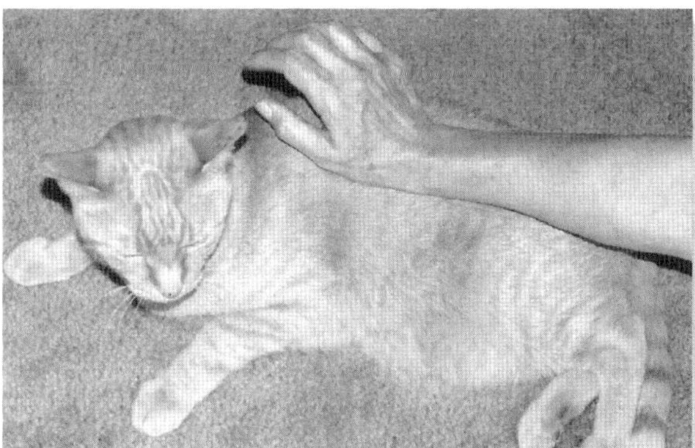

Flat Hand Closing

Perform the Closing exactly the way you began the session: repeat the Opening. By tracing the Bladder meridian with the heel of your hand three times on both sides of your cat, you're again connecting with all the internal organs by virtue of the Association points. The difference is your intention; you are finishing and closing the energy.

You can vary the speed of tracing the Bladder meridian from head to hind fifth digit, depending on how you want to leave the cat. If you want him to be calm, go slowly. If you think the cat's energy needs to be increased, trace the Bladder meridian more quickly.

Post-Session

After the acupressure session, it's important to observe your cat's behavior and watch for any changes in the indicators that were apparent during your original assessment. It takes 24 hours for chi to flow throughout the meridian system, so you may not see any observable changes during the first hours after a session. After the first 24 hours, make special note of any changes. Record these changes so you'll remember the effect your session had on your cat for future sessions.

Wait three to five days before giving your cat another acupressure session. Remember, in the first 24 hours after a session, the chi is rebalancing. The second 24-hour period is when the cat's body is experiencing and adjusting to the shift in energy. On the third day, the effect of the session is more readily seen. This three-to-five day period pertains to a full acupressure session. Sometimes there are specific situations where you only do acupoints and not a complete session.

When does it make sense to offer a cat specific acupoints to deal with a particular issue or situation and not perform a complete session? You can perform acupoint work when you are seeking veterinary attention for an emergency, unconsciousness, calming, and vomiting. These are times when you can help the cat right at that moment. Another good time to offer point work without a full session is post-surgery.

Although there's a lot of complex theory related to acupressure, realize that acupressure works no matter how much or how little theory you know. Chapter Eight provides you with acupressure sessions for 31 common feline conditions. The acupoints selected for each specific condition are based on known attributes of each acupoint. Using these common acupoints is a useful way for beginners to become familiar with points and their energetics and functions.

Acupoints do what they're going to do because of their inherent energetic characteristics and functions. A novice can perform a session that resolves the presenting health issue.

This book guides you through a comprehensive acupressure session. That said, the more you study and increase your knowledge of Traditional Chinese Medicine, the more effective the work you do with your cat will be.

Cats are Cats – Short Acupressure Session

Because cats are cats, offering a comprehensive acupressure session each time you settle into an acupressure time together may not be realistic. Many cats don't like to be handled more than what they think is appropriate. Accept that they know what is best for them.

Given their inherent sense of what they can tolerate at a particular time, be sure to respect their choice. Restraining your cat will not accomplish your intention of helping balance your cat's flow of chi and blood. At times, you'll need to shorten the assessment process and go right to the Point Work segment of the session. Simply by performing the Opening, you have already begun the balancing process.

If your cat indicates he is restless or uninterested in having you perform a complete session, you can go right to the acupoint selection after the Opening Phase. Simply select three or four acupoints you think will support his general health and well-being. For instance, if you deem this a health maintenance session, select a few acupoints from the specific condition charts provided in the next chapter.

Other examples are: if you're concerned about your cat's nasal congestion, select acupoints from the respiratory chart; when your cat is exhibiting anxiety, select acupoints from the chart specifically for anxiety reduction; if you have a senior cat, use acupoints related to aging conditions. Take a minute to review the Specific Feline Conditions in Chapter Eight.

After you have completed the point work you've selected from the specific condition charts, you can go ahead and "Close" your cat. You do this by tracing the Bladder meridian three times on each side of the cat in the same way you did for the Opening at the beginning of the session. Closing draws the cat's energy together after moving it around during the point work.

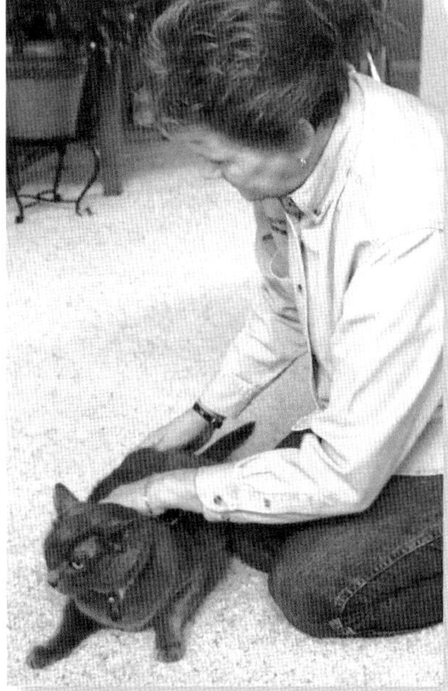
Closing the Bladder meridian

Your cat may have have as much touching as he needs and doesn't want to sit still for the Closing. Not to worry; he'll likely go off and Close his meridians in his own way. Restraining him could result in losing the benefit gained from the rest of the short session.

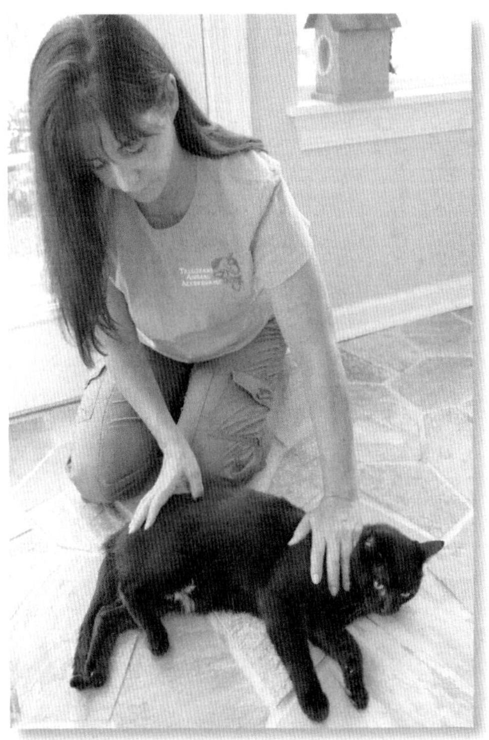

The smallest Feline is a masterpiece.
– Leonardo da Vinci

Chapter Eight

Feline Specific Conditions

A good way to begin your adventure into feline acupressure is to rely on "tried and true" acupoints. Centuries of clinical observation by highly trained Traditional Chinese Medicine doctors brings us a treasure trove of the energetic functions of acupoints. Why not start by working with acupoints known to have energetic attributes intended to resolve a specific condition?

This chapter provides a series of acupressure sessions to address common feline physical and emotional conditions. The acupoints selected for each session have proven to address these specific conditions. Using these points is a place to begin working with your cat once you have performed the assessment process given in Chapters Six and Seven.

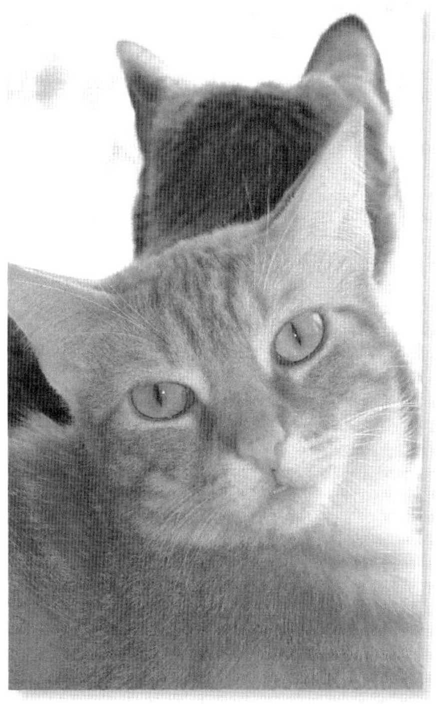

Review the Four Examinations and the functions of the Zang-Fu (internal) organs. Addressing your cat's current condition is essential. And if you feel confident in your assessment, use the Association and Source acupoints that are most directly connected to the organ system related to your cat's pattern of disharmony.

For instance, say that one day Snowman behaves like a "wild and crazy guy" running up the living room drapes and the next day he limps badly. After having him checked by your holistic veterinarian and finding out he has a minor tendon issue, you want to help Snowman's tendon to heal. Remember, Liver and Gall Bladder organ systems are associated with the health of tendons and ligaments.

A basic and effective approach to selecting acupoints is using Bladder 18 (Bl 18), the Association point for the Liver, and Liver 3 (Liv 3), the Source point for the Liver. This helps in your point selection for a session intended to bring more chi and blood to Snowman's tendons. To add more "value" to the session, you can add Gall Bladder 34 (GB 34), the Influential point for tendons and ligaments.

Another approach to the Point Work segment of the session is to rely on acupoints with energetics known to affect the condition your cat is experiencing. This "cookbook" approach can yield a highly effective session especially when you know your cat's issue is arthritis or an ear infection.

Ideally, you will continue to study and learn more about the Zang-Fu organ functions. Being able to identify imbalances of specific organ systems takes time and knowledge. Having specific condition acupoints readily available in this chapter offers you immediate access to the rich resources of Chinese medicine.

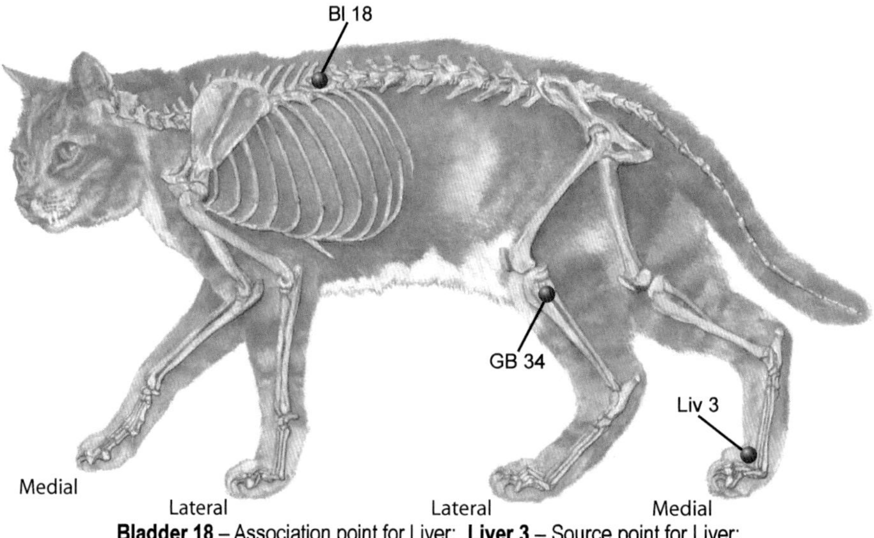

Bladder 18 – Association point for Liver; **Liver 3** – Source point for Liver; **Gall Bladder 34** – Influential point for tendons and ligaments

Remember, chi takes 24 hours to circulate throughout the cat's body. You may not see any change during the first 24-hour cycle. In fact, your cat may seem worse. Don't overreact; this is not uncommon. The animal can appear to be sicker than before, it's known as a "healing crisis." What is actually happening is that the "illness" is moving through his body and is being resolved. Of course, if your cat's condition continues to deteriorate, consult your veterinarian immediately.

Observe your cat for the next two to three days. If your cat is receiving the therapeutic effect you intended, include these same acupoints in your next session. If there's little or no benefit, vary your acupoints based on the organ systems involved or other points suggested in this chapter.

Local and Distal Acupoints

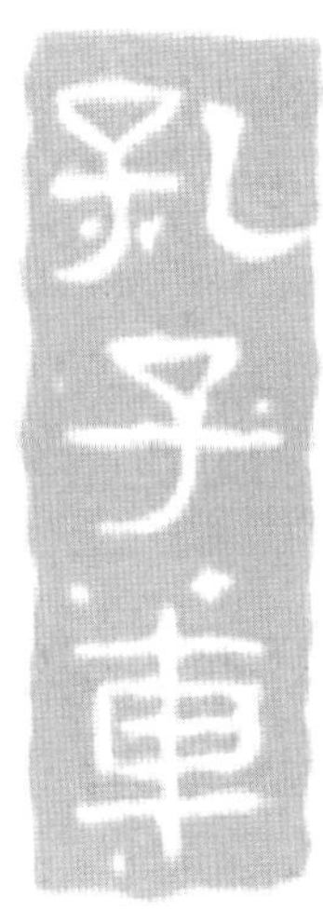

Once you know the location of the 12 Major Meridians and two Extraordinary Vessels, you are able to work with another method of selecting acupoints. That is, you can use acupoints in the vicinity of where the actual problem is located. This is called using "local points" for musculoskeletal issues and specific organ imbalances.

Say Snowman's tendon pain is located on the medial aspect (inside) of his forelimb. His guardian could use acupoints above and below the painful area on his leg where specific meridians are passing through. The Lung, Pericardium, and Heart meridians flow along the medial side of the cat's forelimb. This technique helps move both chi and blood through the injured area.

Using local acupoints is often combined with selecting a "distal" point. A distal acupoint has energetics affecting the area or issue related to the injury. Gall Bladder 34 (GB 34) is considered a distal point for Snowman's tendon injury. GB 34 is located on the hind limb—a distance from the injury site—and has the effect of enhancing the supply of nourishment to his tendons.

Another example of how to use local and distal acupoints is when your cat has conjunctivitis (inflammation of the mucous membrane that lines the exposed portion of the eyeball and inner surface of the eyelids). The local points surrounding the eye are: Bladder 1, Stomach 1, and Gall Bladder 1. The distal point you can include in your point selection is

Liver 2, located on the hind paw. Liver 2 is known to benefit the health and sensory acuity of the eye.

Distal points can come into play when your cat doesn't want you to touch the area that hurts or get anywhere near it. Cats usually communicate clearly about what they're willing to let you do and not do. Better to stay away from the offending location than to have an angry cat, right?

To track down the best distal point for a specific issue, review Chapter Five, the Acupoint Classification chapter. Master points and Influential points function as excellent distal points. If your cat has a drippy nose, Lung 7 (Lu 7)—the Master point for the head and neck—is located on the medial side of the forelimb just above the carpus. Lu 7 is distally located from the cat's nose. Bladder 12, the Influential point for "wind and trachea," supports Lung function and it too, is located a distance from your cat's drippy nose.

At least a hundred methods exist for selecting acupoints for the Point Work part of your acupressure session. Because you have to start somewhere, start where you are comfortable and think you can benefit your cat most. It takes study, understanding, and practice to become proficient at selecting acupoints that address your cat's health and behavior conditions. The key is to start!

The rest of this chapter is devoted to specific feline conditions with acupoints known to benefit these conditions. You don't have to use all of the points on the charts in one session; use only two or three points for your first acupressure session. If those acupoints yield the effect you intend, repeat them in the second session. If not, use other suggested acupoints.

The acupoints given for specific feline conditions in the following pages are general points. The points presented may not address the exact moment in the progression of your cat's current problem nor the root of your cat's health issue. Remember to record your assessment, point selections, observations, and any significant reactions your cat has to the acupressure session for the following 24 to 48-hours post-session.

Feline Aging Issues

As cats age, their Source or essence chi, housed in the Kidney, diminishes until there's too little remaining to sustain life. This is the natural progression of life beginning when the kitten arrives on earth, matures, and then declines over many years. The cat's Zang-Fu organ function slows down as the cat's *Jing*, or essence chi, lessens. The strength and vitality of the cat's overall musculoskeletal structural system decreases as well.

Receiving acupressure, along with eating natural food and living a healthy lifestyle, helps your cat enjoy life for as long as possible. You can do a good job of supporting your cat's Jing; however, aging issues are inevitable.

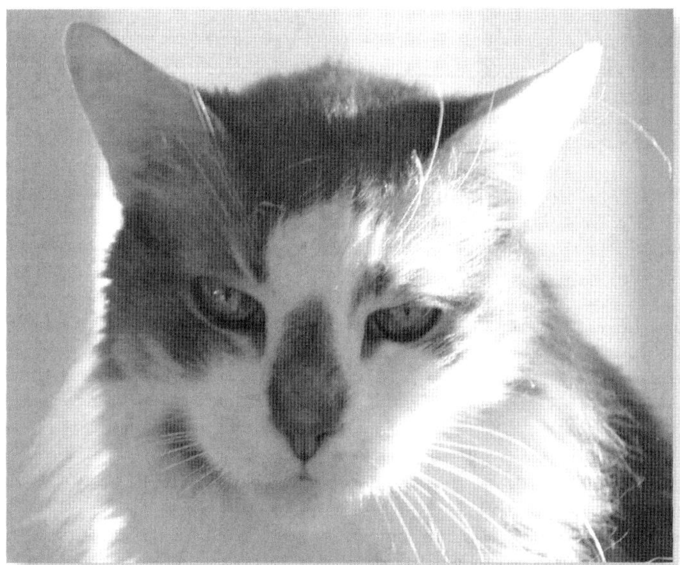

General Aging

Indicators

- Disorientation, loss of memory
- General weakness
- Overall slowing down
- Hindquarter weakness
- Increased sleeping
- Decreased playing

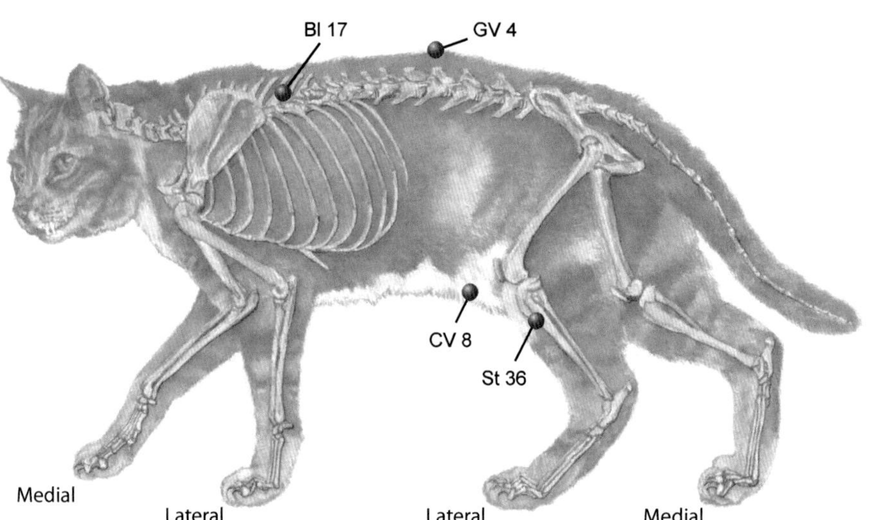

Point	Name	Location
St 36	Leg 3 Miles	Craniolateral aspect of the pelvic limb. One finger-breadth lateral to the tibial crest in the lateral portion of the cranial tibial muscle. 3 cun below St 35.
Bl 17	Diaphragm's Transport	1.5 cun lateral to the caudal border of the spinous process of the 7th thoracic vertebra.
CV 8	Spirit's Palace Gate	On the ventral midline, in the center of the umbilicus.
GV 4	Vital Gate	On the dorsal midline between the spinous processes of the 2nd and 3rd lumbar vertebrae.

Urinary Problems

Indicators

- General loss of urinary control
- Leaking during the night
- Dribbling while heading outside or to litter box

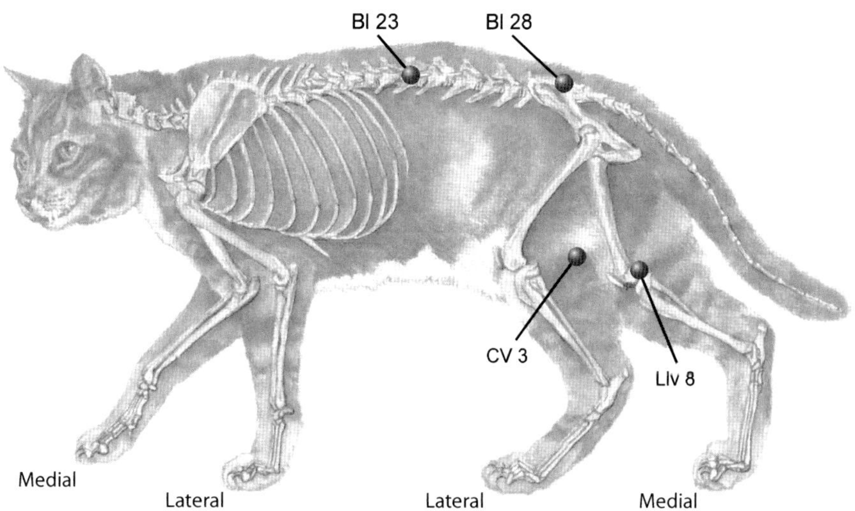

Point	Name	Location
Bl 23	Kidney's Transport	1.5 cun lateral to the spinous process of the 2nd lumbar vertebra.
Bl 28	Bladder's Transport	Lateral to the 2nd foramen, in the depression between the sacrum and the medial border of the dorsal iliac spine.
Liv 8	Curved Spring	In a depression on the medial end of the transverse popliteal crease, between the medial condyle of the femur and the attachment of the semimembranosus muscle.
CV 3	Central Pole	On the ventral midline, 4 cun caudal to the umbilicus.

Arthritis

Arthritis (the deterioration of cartilage and bone) tends to occur as cats age. In TCM, it's basically considered a chronic "cold" condition because of the loss of essential vitality of the bone. Additionally, arthritis is a type of "Bi Syndrome," which is a painful condition characterized by a blockage of chi and blood circulation. More specifically, arthritis, osteoarthritis, and spondylosis are called "Bony Bi Patterns of Disharmony." This pattern is brought about by an invasion of external pathogens such as Wind, Cold, Damp, and Heat. In general, arthritis is a deficiency pattern.

Selecting acupoints for an acupressure session depends on where and how the arthritis manifests. The three most frequently seen arthritic conditions are Worse with Cold, Worse in Wet Weather, and Joints Exhibit Heat. You need to assess how your cat's arthritis presents and then choose the most appropriate points from the chart.

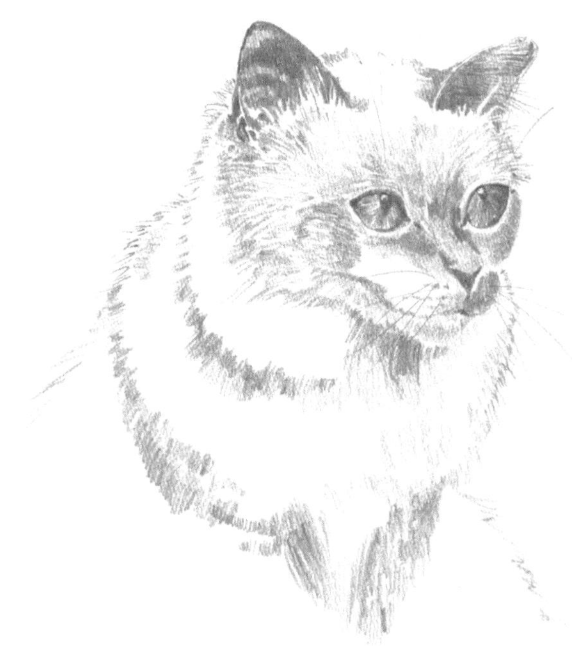

Worse with Cold

Indicators

- Limited mobility
- Intense pain or deep ache
- Arthritic area may feel cold; joints and surrounding muscle may be involved

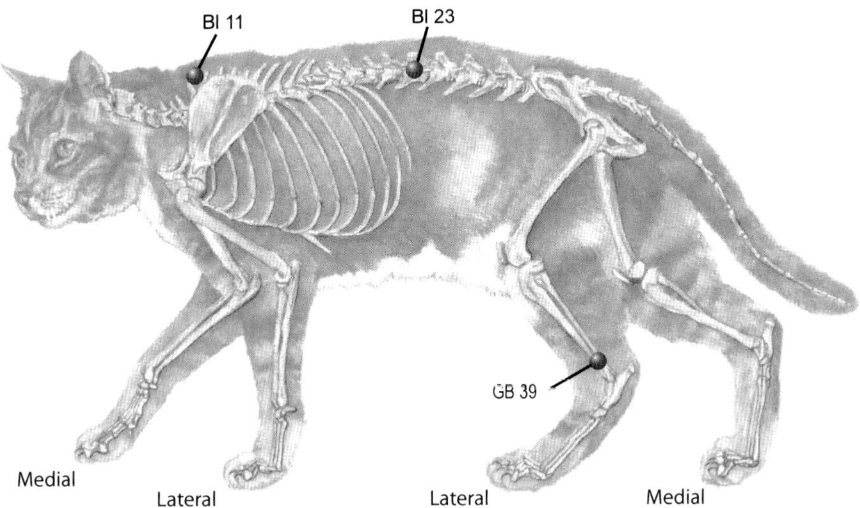

Point	Name	Location
Bl 11	Great Shuttle	1.5 cun lateral to dorsal midline, at cranial edge of the scapula.
Bl 23	Kidney's Transport	1.5 cun lateral to the caudal border of the spinous process of the 2nd lumbar vertebra.
GB 39	Suspended Bell	3 cun above the tip of the lateral malleolus, in depression directly across from Sp 6.

Worse in Wet Weather

Indicators

- Stiff, aching joints
- Possible edema around joint and down leg
- Damp environment increases discomfort

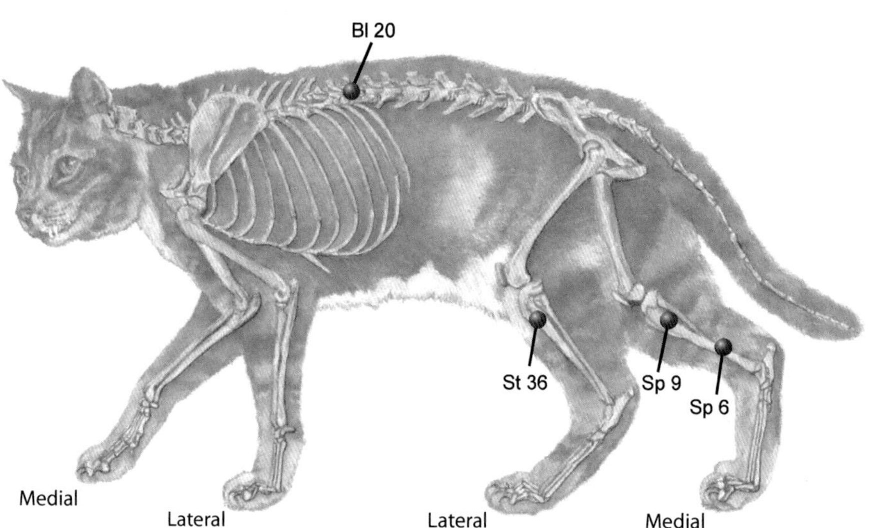

Point	Name	Location
Bl 20	Spleen's Transport	1.5 cun lateral to the spinous process of the 12th thoracic vertebra.
St 36	Leg 3 Miles	Craniolateral aspect of the hind limb. One finger-breadth lateral to the tibial crest in the lateral portion of the cranial tibial muscle. 3 cun below St 35.
Sp 6	3 Yin Meeting	3 cun above the tip of the medial malleolus, on the caudal border of the tibia.
Sp 9	Yin Mound Spring	Medial aspect of the pelvic limb, in a depression between the caudal border of the tibia and gastrocnemius muscle.

Joints Exhibit Heat

Heat is present because of inflammation of the joint tissues. The heat represents an acute occurrence even though the underlying condition is a chronic cold condition in which the bone and cartilage are deteriorating.

Indicators

- Acutely painful (sudden onset)
- Joints are swollen and hot
- Pain increases with pressure
- Minimal mobility

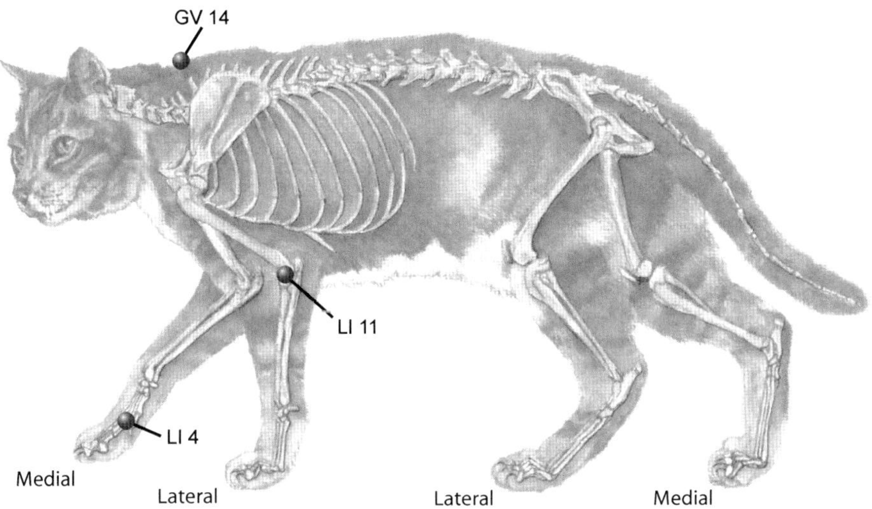

Point	Name	Location
LI 4	Adjoining Valley	Between the 1st (dewclaw) and 2nd metacarpal bones, on the medial side of the 2nd metacarpal.
LI 11	Crooked Pond	Lateral aspect of the thoracic limb. At the lateral end of the cubital crease. Find by flexing the elbow.
GV 14	Big Vertebra	On the dorsal midline between the spinous processes of the last cervical and 1st thoracic vertebrae.

Behavior Issues

Cat behavior can be quixotic, to say the least. At one moment, you're with the most gentle and affectionate being on earth; the next moment, your cat turns into a raging maniac trying to claw your arm to shreds. When that happens, cat people know to let their hand and arm "play dead." Because cats stop being aggressive when they have "killed" their prey, don't try to pull your hand away because your cat will go after a moving hand.

Sudden changes in behavior may not make sense to you, but they must make sense to your cat. There are cat behaviorists who may be able to give you insights into surprising cat behaviors, but most people are just continually surprised.

Feline aggression, for instance, can be based on fear, anger, insecurity, or even a form of play – however misguided it may be. It isn't easy to figure out why cats become aggressive. If your cat's aggression seems related to fear, then Kidney could be involved. If your cat's aggressiveness seems based on anger, the Liver may be imbalanced. And when a cat is defensively aggressive, he could be insecure, which is associated with Stomach and Spleen.

When the aggressive behavior appears to be a game and he's "playing" with you, well, you can attribute this behavior to being "the nature of the beast." Cats are predatory by nature; at that moment, the hand you're petting him with is his idea of a rodent.

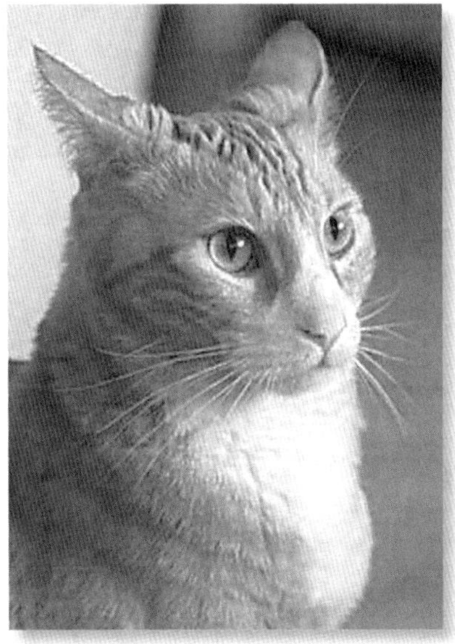

How do you discover why your cat is being aggressive? You need to be acutely aware of the event that seems to provoke his aggressive behavior. Perhaps other indicators can lead you to understanding your cat's motivation. For example, when a cat is defensive and insecure, he may also have trouble digesting his food. Cats feeling afraid tend to respond to situations inconsistently—sometimes by being aggressive and other times by hiding. An angry cat expresses aggression clearly, often as a reaction to current or past torment.

In addition, living among humans can be stressful for cats. As our close companions, they witness our behavior and absorb our emotions.

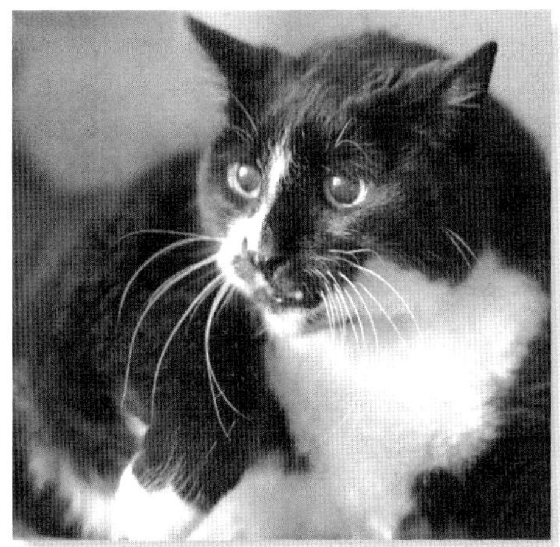

Other stressful situations include not getting enough exercise and not having enough social interaction or mental stimulation. Also, because cats are territorial, moving to a new house or remodeling an existing house can challenge and stress them. So can adding a new pet or human to the household. Any change in routine can trigger a cat's inability to cope.

According to TCM, chronic stress can lead to a shen, or spirit disturbance, which can result in heart-related issues. If a shen disturbance is endured for a long time, it can manifest physically and involve a number of organ systems.

When you're selecting acupoints for a session, it's critical to observe your cat's behavior and take note of the surrounding situation and environment. What triggers precede the behavior? Use your observations as well as your intuition to sort the relevant behavioral cues your cat responds to, and then select points from the following common behavioral issues.

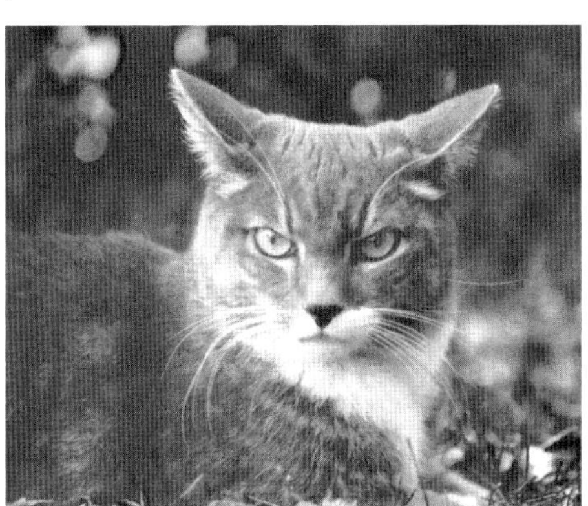

Aggression

Indicators

- Inappropriate biting
- Extreme domination
- Initiating fights
- Pouncing
- Irascibility
- Fear/apprehension

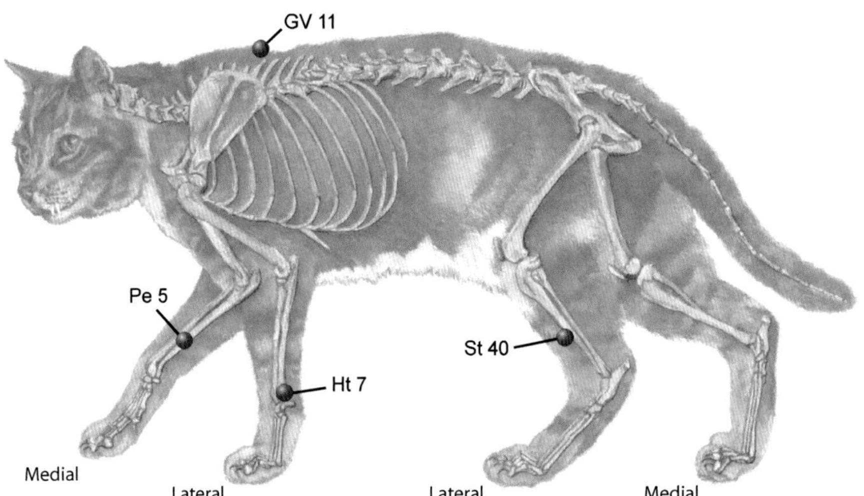

Point	Name	Location
St 40	Abundant Flourishing	Halfway between the lateral malleolus of the fibula and the top of the tibia, on the lateral aspect of the hind leg.
Ht 7	Spirit's Gate	Found at transverse crease of the carpal joint, in a depression lateral to the flexor carpi ulnaris. Opposite Pe 7.
Pe 5	Intermediary	4 cun above the transverse carpal crease, in the muscle groove, on the medial aspect of the thoracic limb.
GV 11	Spirit's Path	In the depression between the dorsal spinous process of the 5th and 6th thoracic vertebrae, on the dorsal midline.

Stress / Anxiety

Indicators

- Compulsive behaviors
- Destructive behaviors
- Self-mutilation
- Chaotic behavior
- Inappropriate urination / defecation / spraying

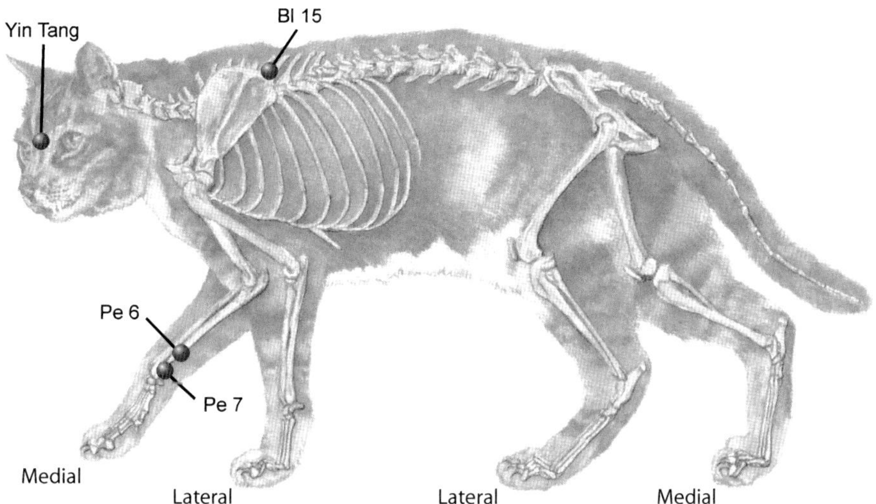

Point	Name	Location
Bl 15	Heart's Transport	1.5 cun lateral to the caudal border of the 5th thoracic vertebra.
Pe 6	Inner Gate	2 cun above the transverse crease of the carpus (wrist), between the tendons of the superficial digital flexors.
Pe 7	Big Mound	Found caudal to the tendon of the flexor carpi radialis and directly above the carpal bone.
Yin Tang		Found on the dorsal midline, just above the level of the eyes.

Fear

Indicators

- Submissive posturing
- Submissive urination / spraying
- Running away or hiding
- Hissing and/or biting

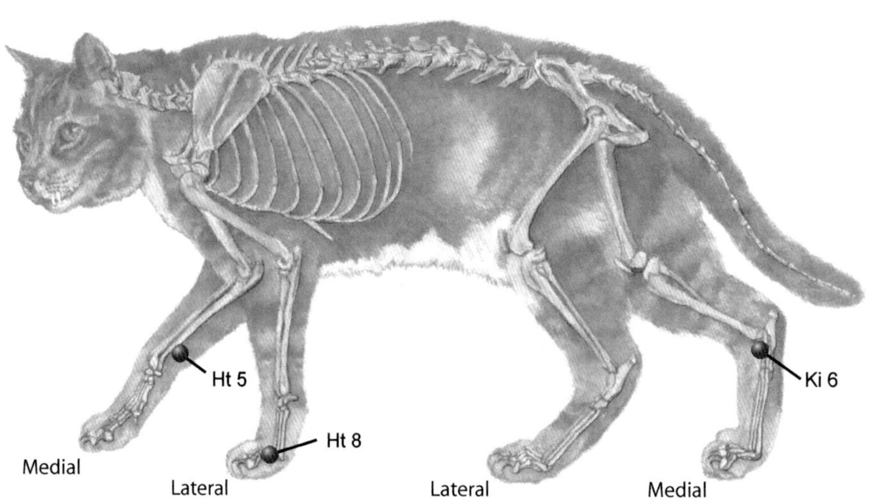

Point	Name	Location
Ht 5	Communication's Route	On the caudal aspect of the forelimb, 1.5 cun above the carpus.
Ht 8	Lesser Palace	Between the 4th and 5th metacarpal bones, just above the metacarpal pad.
Ki 6	Luminous Sea	On the medial aspect of the hind limb, in a depression just below and behind the medial malleolus.

Grief

Indicators

- Refusal to eat
- No interest in playing
- Lethargic disposition
- Lackluster eyes
- Depression / sadness

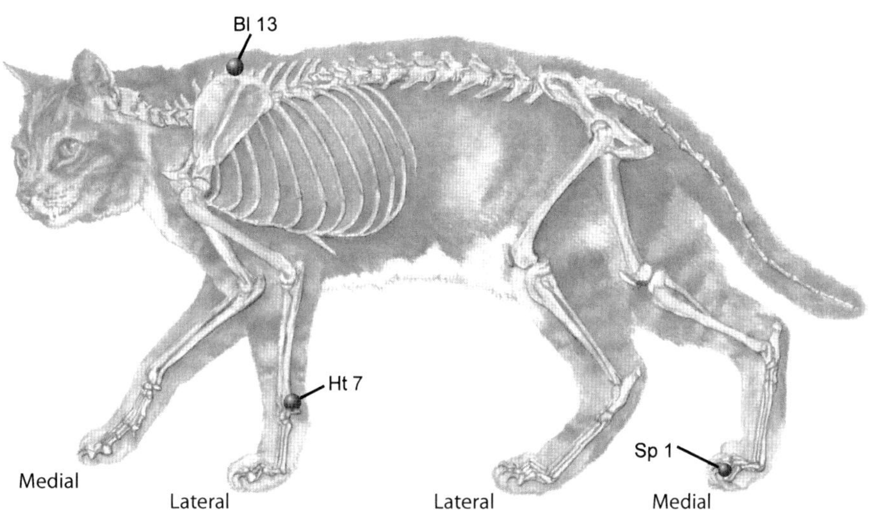

Point	Name	Location
Sp 1	Hidden Clarity	On the medial side of the 2nd digit of the hind paw, at the nail bed.
Ht 7	Spirit's Gate	On lateral side of the transverse crease of the carpal joint, opposite Pe 7.
Bl 13	Lung's Transport	1.5 cun lateral to caudal border of the dorsal spinous process of the 3rd thoracic vertebra.

Stress Reactions

Indicators

- Aggression
- Hiding
- Erratic or sudden change in behavior
- Litter box avoidance
- Inappropriate urination or spraying
- Loss of appetite
- Compulsive grooming
- Loss of hair (psychogenic alopecia)
- Depression
- Physical illness

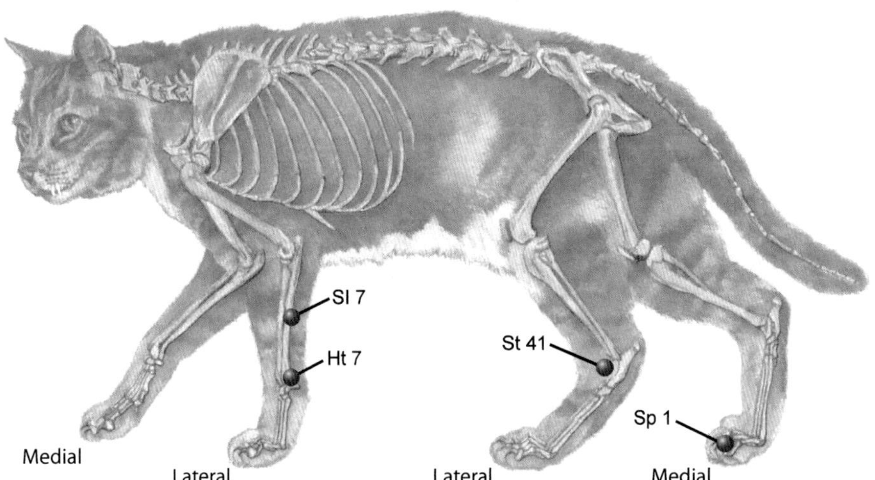

Point	Name	Location
St 41	Release Stream	On the cranial aspect of hock in a depression on the midline, at the level of the lateral malleolus.
Sp 1	Hidden Clarity	On the medial side of the 2nd digit of the hind paw, at the nail bed.
Ht 7	Spirit's Gate	On lateral side of the transverse crease of the carpal joint, opposite Pe 7.
SI 7	Branch to Heart	Lateral aspect of the forelimb about 5/12ths the distance from the carpus to the cubital fossa.

Gastrointestinal Disorders

Consult your holistic veterinarian when your cat experiences gastrointestinal difficulty. Having diarrhea even for a short time can lead to dehydration, especially in a small cat body. Excessive vomiting could indicate a host of health issues including poisoning. A gastric blockage, also called bloat, requires immediate veterinary attention because it's often fatal.

Yes, cats often cough up hairballs, also called "trichobezoars." The coughing sounds awful and the retching seems painful, but it isn't. Cats, especially long-haired cats, can ingest a lot of hair during their grooming regime. They have to regurgitate the hair in a tubular wad so that it doesn't go further down the gastrointestinal tract and cause a dangerous blockage. Usually, cats are good at eliminating their hairballs, but watch your cat in case he can't rid himself of a hairball easily. Indicators include excessive nonproductive gagging/retching, constipation, lethargy, not eating, and constipation or diarrhea.

How can you assist your cat in lessening the formation of hairballs? By brushing him. In addition, you can purchase natural products that will help him rid himself of hairballs quickly and easily.

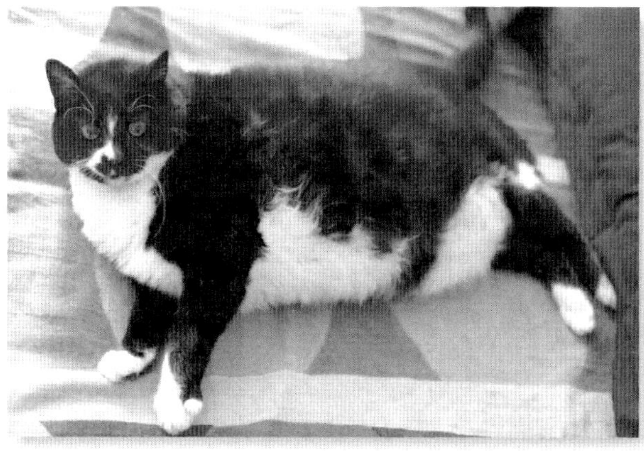

Constipation / Diarrhea

Indicators (Constipation)

- Difficult, infrequent, or absent bowel movement
- Loss of appetite
- Dehydration
- Abdominal distention and pain

Indicators (Diarrhea)

- Soft, loose, or watery stools
- Larger than usual stools
- Mucous in stools
- Frequent excretion

Note: the acupoints are the same for Constipation and Diarrhea because both are an imbalance of the digestive process and these acupoints help to restore balance.

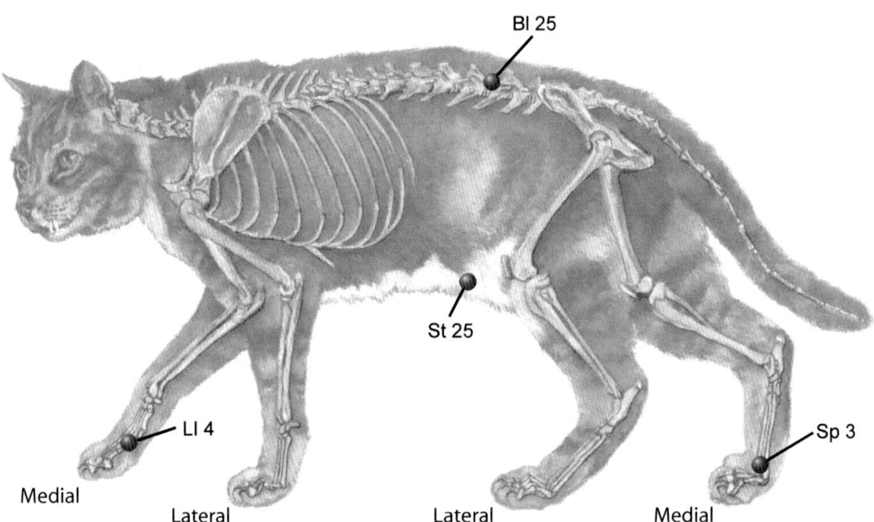

Point	Name	Location
LI 4	Adjoining Valley	Between the 1st (dewclaw) and 2nd metacarpal bones, on the medial side of the 2nd metacarpal.
St 25	Heavenly Pillar	Found 2 cun lateral to the umbilicus.
Sp 3	Great Whiteness	Medial aspect of hindleg above the metatarsophalangeal joint on medial side of 2nd metatarsal bone.
Bl 25	Lg Intestine Transport	1.5 cun lateral to the spinous process of the 5th lumbar vertebra.

Indigestion

Indicators

- Vomiting
- Weight loss
- Increased attempts to defecate with less production
- Increased mucous or blood in stool
- Exercise intolerance
- Hot ears or nose
- Weakness or stiffness of the hindquarters

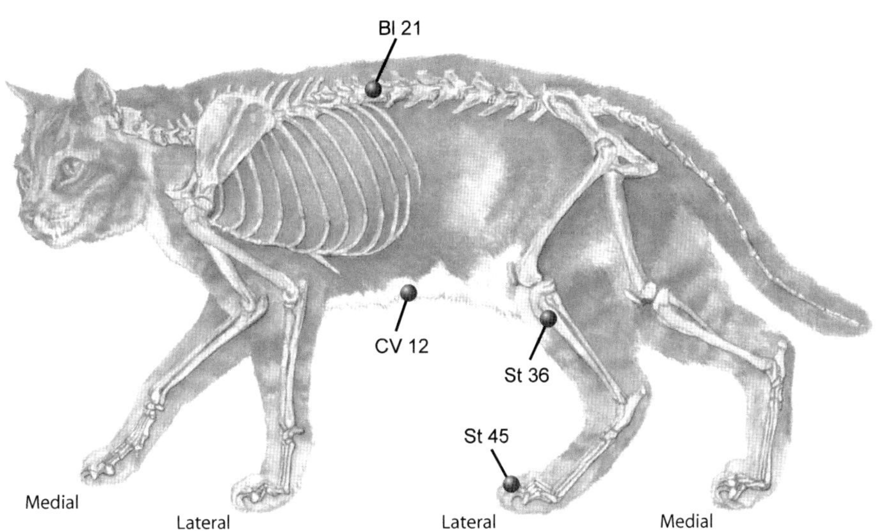

Point	Name	Location
St 36	Leg 3 Miles	Craniolateral aspect of the pelvic limb. One finger-breadth lateral to the tibial crest in the lateral portion of the cranial tibial muscle. 3 cun below St 35.
St 45	Evil's Dissipation	On the lateral side of the 3rd digit of the hind paw, at the nail bed.
Bl 21	Stomach's Transport	1.5 cun lateral to the spinous process of the 13th thoracic vertebra.
CV 12	Sea of Power	On the ventral midline, halfway between the xiphoid process and the umbilicus.

Vomiting

Stomach chi is supposed to descend. However, when it ascends, it causes vomiting, which is called "Rebellious Stomach chi." Overeating, shen disturbances, or exogenous pathogens commonly lead to vomiting of food.

NOTE: The hair ingested during your cat's careful grooming forms a ball in his stomach that needs to be expelled. Regurgitating a hairball is absolutely necessary to avoid an intestinal blockage. Don't interfere with your cat's efforts to rid himself of hairballs.

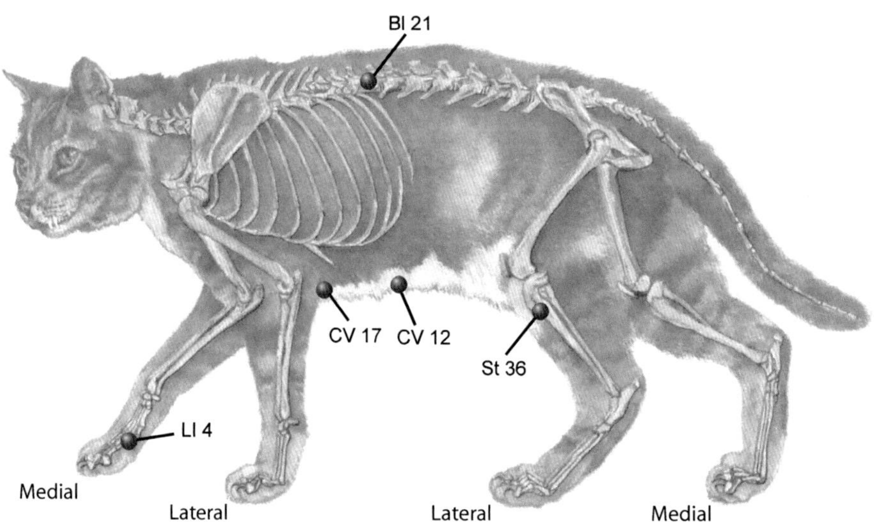

Point	Name	Location
LI 4	Adjoining Valley	Between the 1st (dewclaw) and 2nd metacarpal bones, on the medial side of the 2nd metacarpal.
St 36	Leg 3 Miles	Craniolateral aspect of the pelvic limb. One finger-breadth lateral to the tibial crest in the lateral portion of the cranial tibial muscle. 3 cun below St 35.
Bl 21	Stomach's Transport	1.5 cun lateral to the caudal border of the spinous process of the 13th thoracic vertebra.
CV 12	Sea of Power	On the ventral midline, halfway between the xiphoid process and the umbilicus.
CV 17	Sea of Tranquility	On the ventral midline, at the level of the caudal border of the 4th intercostal space.

Immune System Strengthening

There's no cat alive that doesn't need an Immune System Strengthening acupressure session regularly. Cats are constantly contending with airborne and material toxins in their environment. Those living in urban, suburban, and rural areas are constantly exposed to chemicals from many sources. These toxins include metals in the air, chemical cleaners in the home, and fertilizers or biocides on plants or in the soil. All of these toxins compromise your cat's immune system.

When Defensive or *Wei* chi is weak, the immune system will be weak or compromised. That means external or internal pathogenic factors disrupt the balance of the body. The organ systems that most affect the immune system are the Lungs, Kidneys, and Liver organ systems. Acupoints, shown in the following chart, strengthen the immune system:

- **Lung 7** – Stimulates the descending and dispersing of Lung chi and Defensive chi
- **Large Intestine 4** – Tonifies chi flow and Defensive chi
- **Stomach 36** – Tonifies chi and blood and strengthens the body
- **Spleen 6** – Nourishes blood and yin, promotes the function of the Liver and Liver chi
- **Bladder 23** – Supports and nourishes the Kidneys and kidney essence, nourishes blood
- **Governing Vessel 14** – Regulates Nutritive and Defensive chi, builds yang

To help your cat cope with every day, mild stress and environmental toxins, offer him an Immune System Strengthening session weekly. The acupoints given in the chart can be used for a general health maintenance session as well as following any surgery, trauma, and vaccination.

Immune System Issues

Indicators

- Frequent or chronic infections or illness
- Slow healing of superficial wounds
- Exhibiting allergic conditions (eye or nasal discharge, chronic skin problems)
- Exposure to animals with contagious conditions
- Reactions to medications including vaccinations
- Exposure to toxins

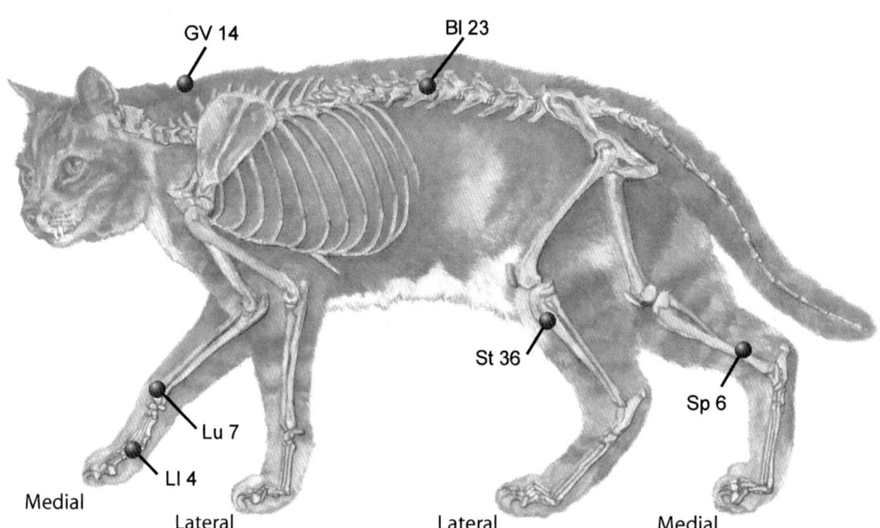

Point	Name	Location
Lu 7	Broken Sequence	Proximal to the styloid process of the radius, 1.5 cun above the transverse crease of the carpus.
LI 4	Adjoining Valley	Between the 1st (dewclaw) and 2nd metacarpal bones, on the medials side of the 2nd matacarpal.
St 36	Leg 3 Miles	Craniolateral aspect of the pelvic limb. One finger-breadth lateral to the tibial crest in the lateral portion of the cranial tibial muscle. 3 cun below St 35.
Sp 6	3 Yin Meeting	3 cun above the tip of the medial malleolus, on the caudal border of the tibia.
Bl 23	Kidney's Transport	1.5 cun lateral to the caudal border of the spinous process of the 2nd lumbar vertebra.
GV 14	Big Vertebra	On the dorsal midline between the spinous processes of the last cervical and 1st thoracic vertebrae.

Musculoskeletal Issues

The term "musculoskeletal" refers to the system containing the striated muscles (not the smooth or cardiac muscles) and the skeleton. Issues like arthritis that are related to the musculoskeletal system are called Bi Syndromes. The stiffness and pain associated with these patterns are attributed to the stagnation or blockage of blood and chi within the cat's meridian system. In TCM, this type of pain is linked to an invasion of pathogens such as Wind, Cold, Damp, or Heat. Possibly, a combination of these pathogens are the root of the obstruction of blood and chi.

Although musculoskeletal issues are most often seen in older cats, younger cats can show signs of these issues due to illness, injury, surgical procedures, poor breeding, and poor quality food.

Cats that have musculoskeletal issues tend to hold themselves rigidly in the "sick-cat position." That means their legs are tucked under their bodies, their eyes are squinty or closed, and they are reluctant to move at all. In fact, moving hurts. If your cat gives evidence of not wanting to move or any musculoskeletal problems, it's wise to have a vet check him before performing an acupressure session.

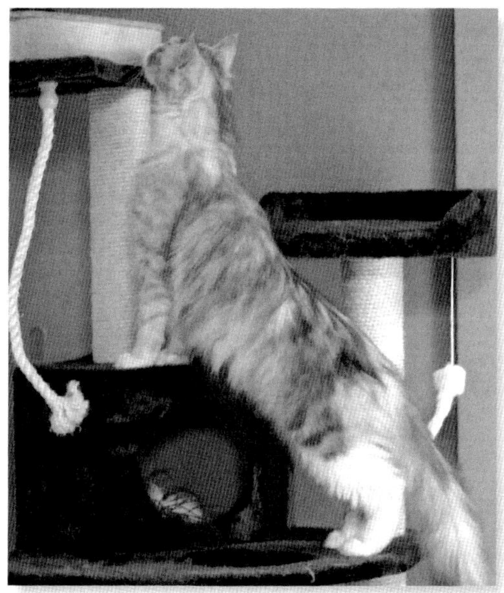

Cervical / Neck Issues

Indicators

- Restricted or painful neck movement
- Unusual or inappropriate head carriage
- Difficulty raising or lowering the head
- Inability to groom the back
- Swelling

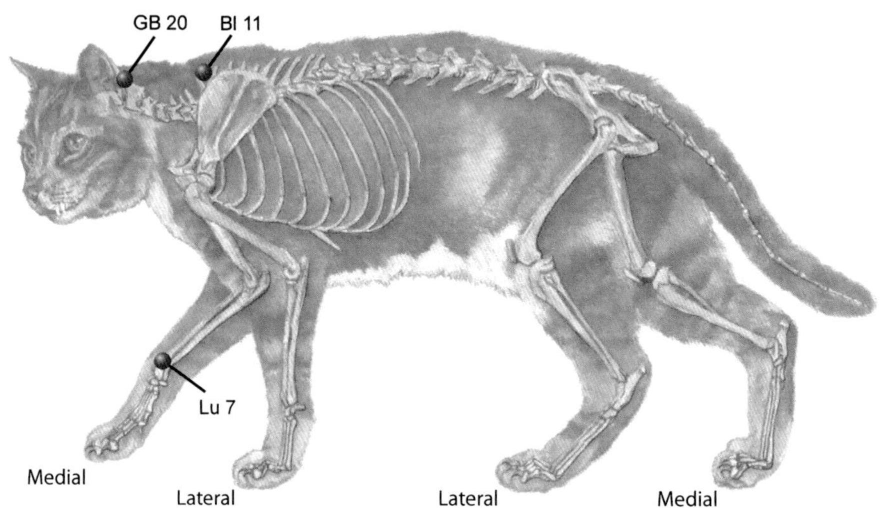

Point	Name	Location
Lu 7	Broken Sequence	Found proximal to the styloid process on the radius, 1.5 cun above the transverse crease of the carpus.
Bl 11	Wind's Gate	1.5 cun lateral to the dorsal midline, at the cranial edge of the scapula.
GB 20	Wind Pool	On the neck, caudal to the occipital bone, in a depression between the occipital bone and wing of the atlas.

Back Soreness

Indicators

- Resistance to touch or brushing
- Difficulty climbing or descending stairs
- Difficulty lying down, sitting, or getting up
- Swelling
- Uneven gait
- Inability to groom himself

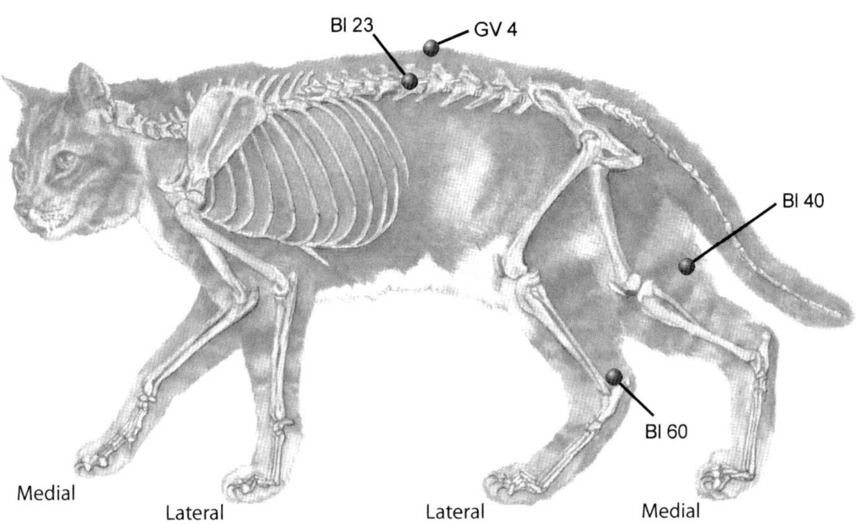

Point	Name	Location
Bl 23	Kidney's Transport	1.5 cun lateral to the spinous process of the 2nd lumbar vertebra.
Bl 40	Supporting the Middle	Located at the midpoint of the transverse crease of the popliteal fossa.
Bl 60	Kunlun Mountain	On the lateral aspect of the hindleg, at the thinnest fleshy tissue of the hock, opposite Ki 3.
GV 4	Vital Gate	On the dorsal midline between the spinous processes of the 2nd and 3rd lumbar vertebrae.

Hip Dysplasia

Unfortunately, the incidence of hip dysplasia in cats is increasing because of poor breeding practices and poor quality, manufactured foods.

Indicators

- Restricted hind limb mobility (lameness)
- Reluctance or refusal to jump
- Loss of interest in playing or running
- Difficulty lying down, sitting, or getting up
- Hindquarter stiffness
- Sensitivity to touch
- Lying down often

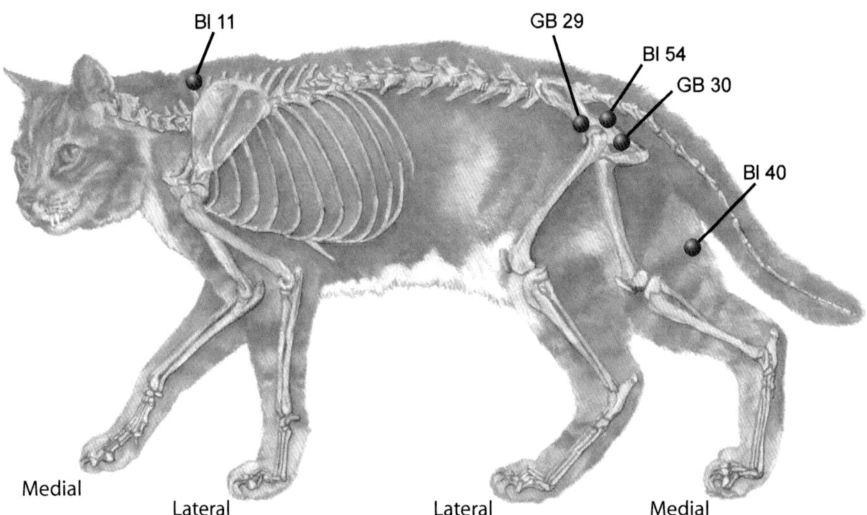

Point	Name	Location
Bl 11	Great Shuttle	1.5 cun lateral to dorsal midline, at cranial edge of the scapula.
Bl 40	Supporting Middle	At midpoint of the transverse crease of the popliteal fossa.
Bl 54	Order's Frontier	Just above (dorsal to) the greater trochanter of the femur.
GB 29	Inhabited Joint	At the coxofemoral joint in the depression cranial to the greater trochanter of the femur.
GB 30	Leaping Circumflexus	Halfway between the greater trochanter of the femur and the tuber ischii.

Shoulder Soreness

Indicators

- Forelimb lameness (limping)
- Difficulty changing directions or turning
- Difficulty in slowing down or stopping
- Difficulty in going up or down stairs
- Lying down constantly

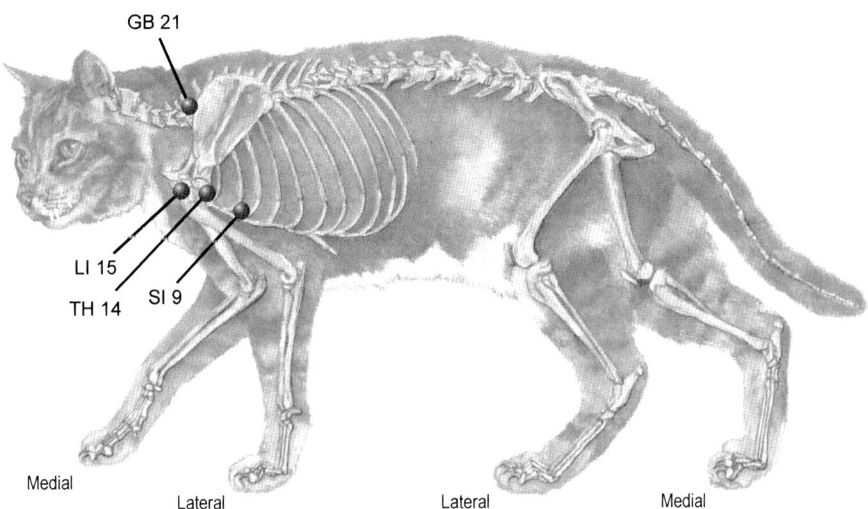

Point	Name	Location
LI 15	Shoulder's Corner	At shoulder region, at the cranial edge of the acromion.
SI 9	Shoulder Integrity	In depression behind the humerus, at the level of the shoulder joint.
TH 14	Shoulder Opening	Behind the acromion of the scapula, on the deltoid muscle.
GB 21	Shoulder Well	Just in front of the scapula, between the 7th cervical and 1st thoracic vertebrae.

Respiratory Conditions

Consult your veterinarian when your cat presents with any feline respiratory distress. Indicators of respiratory issues can range from mild to severe. Even if your cat's indicators seem mild, it's necessary to have him checked immediately. After all, breathing is essential to life.

Cats can experience a host of respiratory illnesses such as asthma, bronchitis, lung and sinus congestion, pneumonia, lung parasites, tumors, and various viruses. Their breathing can become obstructed quickly because of the small size of their respiratory passages.

In TCM, the Lung is thought to be the most vulnerable of the organ systems to external pathogens. When airborne pathogens enter the body, Lung function can be compromised. The Lung plays an extremely important role in the strength of the immune system. Defensive, or *Wei* chi, is based on the proper functioning of the Lung.

In addition, the Lung is responsible for descending chi; the Kidney must be strong enough to grasp the Lung chi and "root the breath." As cats age, the relationship between the Lung and Kidney tends to weaken. Older animals don't breathe as deeply; their breath can be shallow and soft. However, the relationship between Lung and Kidney sustains life until the very last exhale.

A general approach to respiratory issues is to maintain a strong immune system. (Refer to the Immune System Strengthening specific condition included in this chapter to ward off susceptibility to illness.) However, when your cat exhibits a respiratory condition, using acupoints that directly support Lung function will help your cat. The acupressure sessions on the following pages can be administered in conjunction with your veterinarian's recommendations.

Indicators of Respiratory Conditions

Indicators

- Sneezing
- Wheezing
- Hacking/choking/coughing
- Labored breathing
- Gurgling or rattling sound
- Gasping for breath
- Open mouth breathing
- Discharge from nose and eyes
- Choking up foam
- Blue lips, tongue, or gums
- Lethargy or weakness
- Fever
- Loss of appetite

General Lung Support

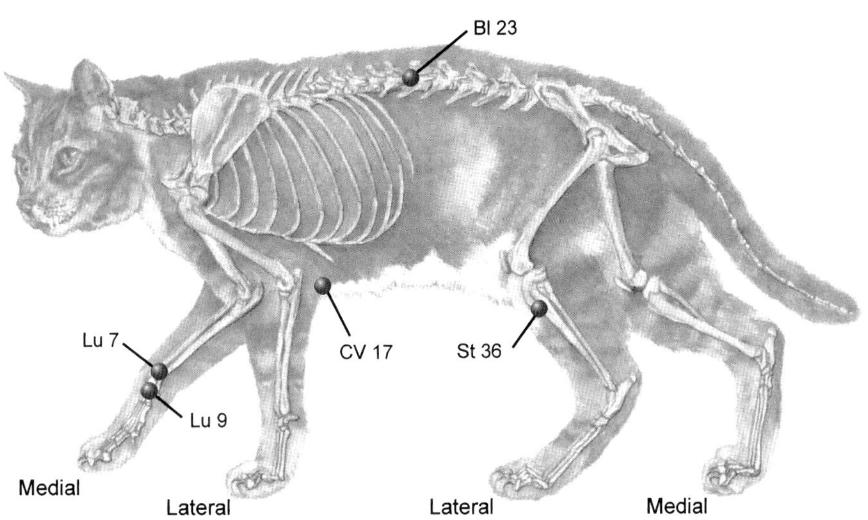

Point	Name	Location
Lu 7	Broken Sequence	Proximal to the styloid process on the radius, 1.5 cun above the transverse crease of the carpus.
Lu 9	Greater Abyss	On the medial aspect of the radiocarpal joint just cranial to (in front of) the radial artery, at the level of Ht 7.
St 36	Leg 3 Miles	Craniolateral aspect of the hind limb. One finger-breadth lateral to the tibial crest in the lateral portion of the cranial tibial muscle. 3 cun below St 35.
Bl 23	Kidney's Transport	1.5 cun lateral to the caudal border of the spinous process of the 2nd lumbar vertebra.
CV 17	Sea of Tranquility	On the ventral midline, at the level of the caudal border of the elbow, about the 4th intercostal space.

Bronchitis

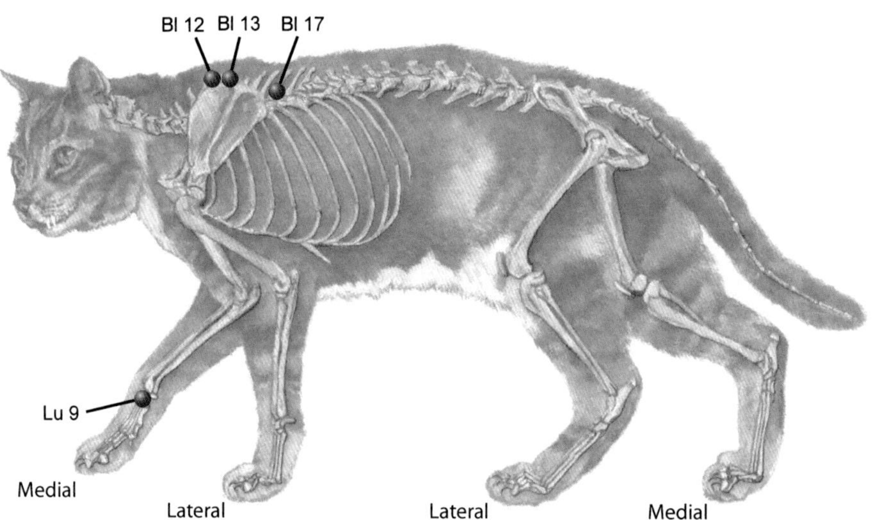

Point	Name	Location
Lu 9	Great Abyss	Located on the medial aspect of the radiocarpal joint, just cranial to the radial artery, at the level of Ht 7.
Bl 12	Wind's Door	1.5 cun lateral to the caudal border of the dorsal spinous process of the 2nd thoracic vertebra.
Bl 13	Lung's Transport	1.5 cun lateral to the caudal border of the dorsal spinous process of the 3rd thoracic vertebra.
Bl 17	Diaphragm's Transport	1.5 cun lateral to the caudal border of the spinous process of the 7th thoracic vertebra.

Asthma

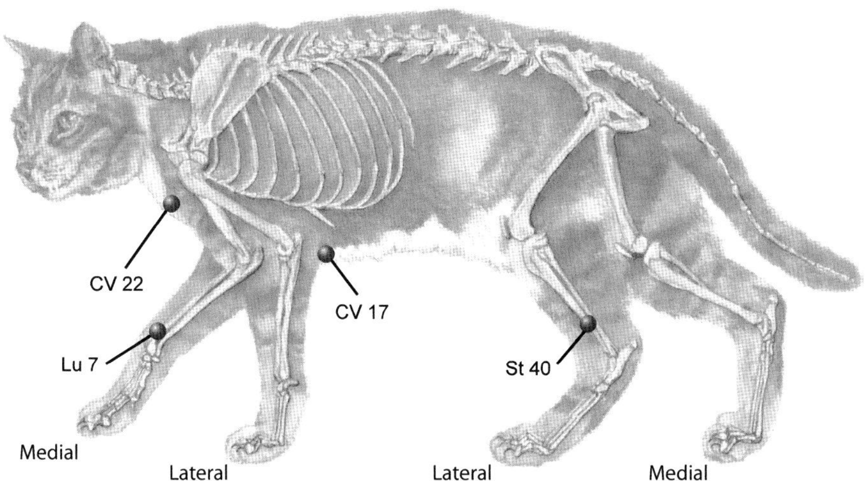

Point	Name	Location
Lu 7	Broken Sequence	Found proximal to the styloid process on the radius, 1.5 cun above the transverse crease of the carpus.
St 40	Abundant Bulge	Located halfway between the lateral malleolus of the fibula and the top of the tibia, on the lateral aspect of the pelvic limb.
CV 17	Sea of Tranquility	On the ventral midline, at the level of the caudal border of the elbow, at the 4th intercostal space.
CV 22	Heaven's Projection	Found on the ventral midline at the tip of the manubrium.

Sensory Issues

With any type of sensory perception, acupressure can help manage and even retard the progression of sensory loss. If you suspect your cat is experiencing a hearing loss or loss of visual acuity, have your holistic veterinarian evaluate his condition. If there's infection, discharge, or heat present, consult a veterinarian immediately.

Ear Infection

Indicators

- Excessive ear scratching
- Heat in or around ear(s)
- Unpleasant odor
- No interest in play

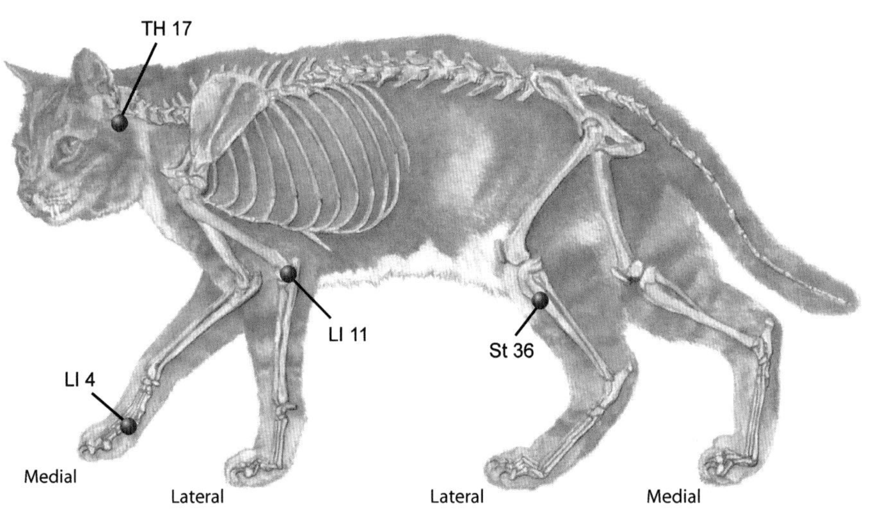

Point	Name	Location
LI 4	Adjoining Valley	Between the 1st (dewclaw) and 2nd metacarpal bones, on the medial side of the 2nd metacarpal.
LI 11	Crooked Pool	Lateral aspect of the thoracic limb, at the lateral end of the cubital crease. Find by flexing the elbow.
St 36	Leg 3 Miles	Craniolateral aspect of the hind limb. One finger-breadth lateral to the tibial crest in the lateral portion of the cranial tibial muscle. 3 cun below St 35.
TH 17	Shielding Wind	Located behind and below the base of the ear.

Hearing Loss

Indicators

- Non-responsive to loud noise
- Ear pain
- Ear Infection

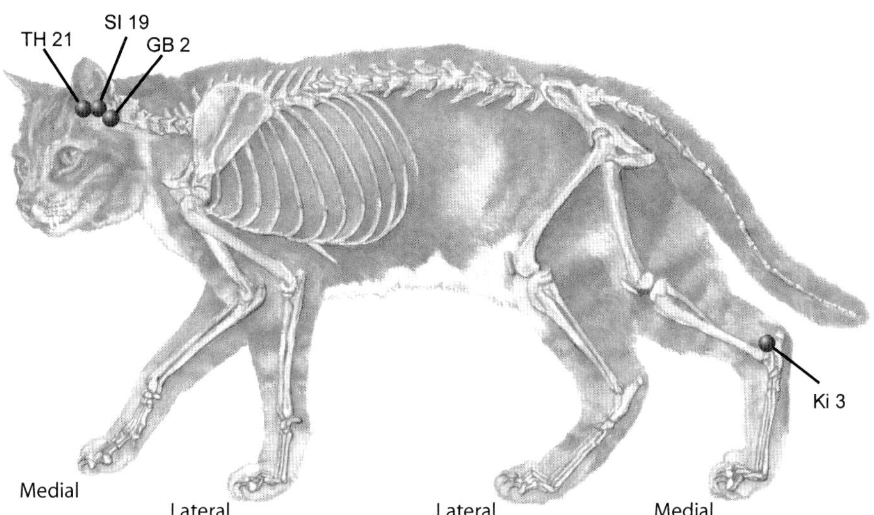

Point	Name	Location
SI 19	Palace of Hearing	In the depression rostral (toward the nose) to the tragus (projection at base of external ear) of the ear.
TH 21	Ear's Gate	In a depression above the condyloid process of the mandible and slightly above SI 19.
GB 2	Reunion of Hearing	About 1.5 cun caudoventral to SI 19, when the mouth is open, there is a depression.
Ki 3	Great Stream	In the depression between the medial malleolus of the tibia and the calcaneal tendon. Opposite Bl 60.

Visual Acuity

Indicators

- Reluctance to engage in activity
- Using other senses to navigate
- Squinting
- Non-responsive to visual cues

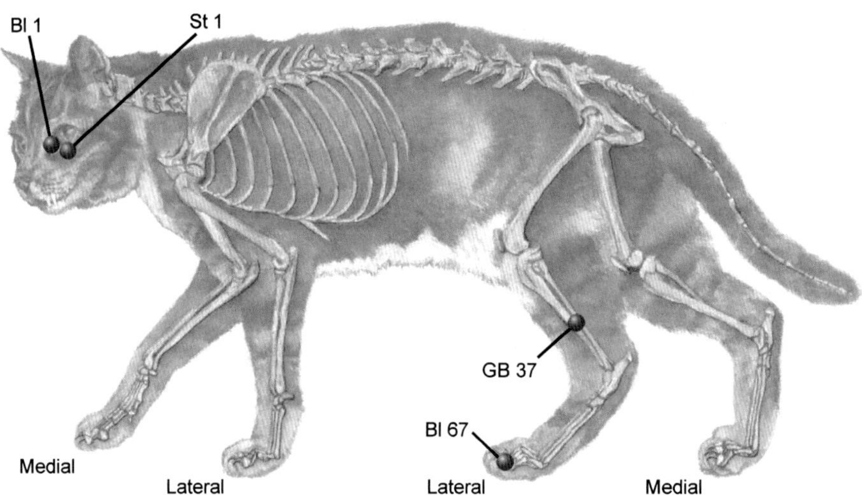

Point	Name	Location
St 1	Containing Tears	Directly below (ventral to) the center of the pupil.
Bl 1	Eye's Clarity	In the indentation dorsal to the medial canthus of the eye.
Bl 67	Reaching Yin	Located on the lateral aspect of the 5th digit of the hind paw, at the nail bed.
GB 37	Bright Light	Located 5 cun above the tip of the lateral malleolus on the anterior border of the fibula.

Conjunctivitis

Indicators

- Severe redness of the lining of the eyelids (conjunctiva)
- Discharge from the eyes *
- Sticky eyelids
- Squinting
- Rubbing of eyes

Clear discharge often indicates an allergic reaction. Yellow or green discharge can indicate infection.

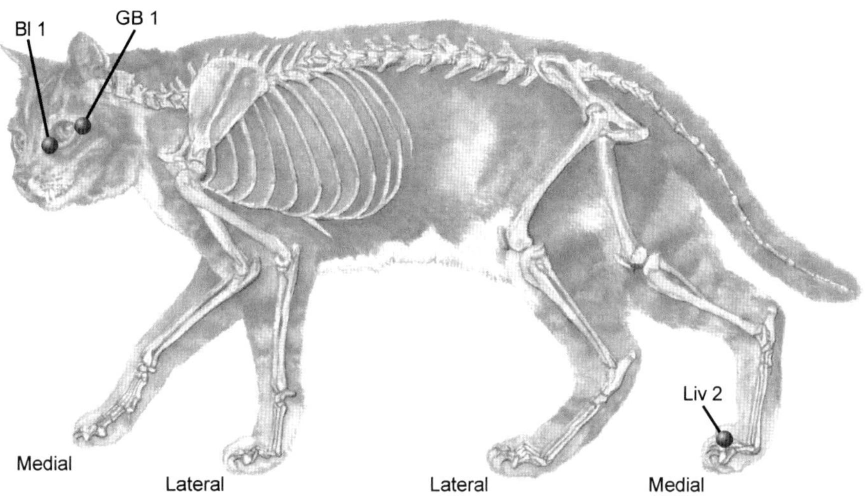

Point	Name	Location
Bl 1	Eye's Clarity	In the indentation dorsal to the medial canthus of the eye.
GB 1	Pupil's Seam	In the depression just lateral to the outer canthus of the eye above the orbital rim.
Liv 2	Travel Between	Distal to the metatarsal phalangeal joint, on the lateral side of the 2nd digit.

Skin Conditions

Cats are susceptible to a long list of skin problems such as bacterial, fungal, or other infections, contact or miliary dermatitis, allergies (airborne or ingested), parasites, acne, alopecia, cancer, etc. Because many skin problems have underlying conditions, your holistic veterinarian is a good resource for identifying the issue and providing topical applications to help resolve your cat's discomfort.

Skin allergies in cats are common. Exposure to household cleaners, pesticides, fertilizers, and other topical irritants can damage their skin. If it seems to be an allergic reaction (such as to a vaccination or an insect bite), go back to the Immune System Strengthening chart, select two to three acupoints, and monitor your cat's response to a session. Within three days, you will know if your cat is improving. If you see no improvement, select another set of two to three points. Continue working in this way to strengthen your cat's general immune system. Please see your veterinarian if your cat doesn't show any improvement.

In TCM, dry, itchy skin is usually attributed to a blood deficiency. That means blood is not nourishing and moistening the skin. The objective of this acupressure session is to enhance the circulation and nourishing quality of blood while supporting the Lung's capacity to disperse blood and chi to the surface of the body.

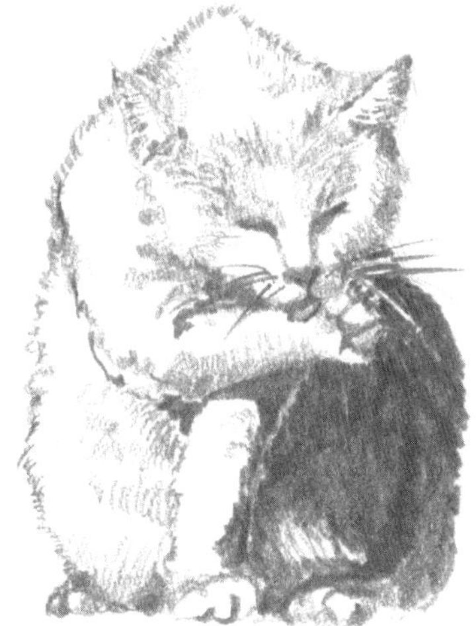

Dry, Itchy Skin

Indicators

- Excessive scratching
- Loss of hair
- Excessive dander
- Brittle, dry coat, lackluster condition

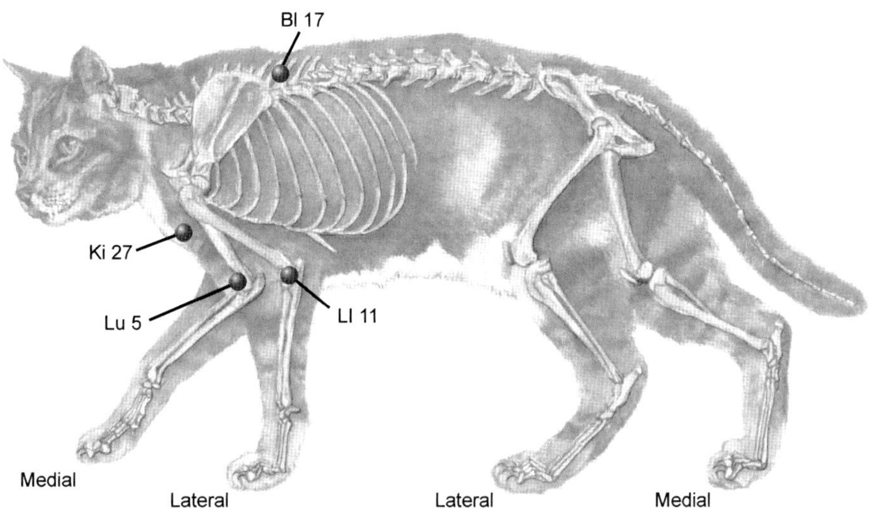

Point	Name	Location
Lu 5	Cubit Marsh	In cubital crease lateral to the tendon of the biceps brachii muscle and medial to the tendon of the brachialis muscle.
LI 11	Crooked Pool	Located on the lateral aspect of the thoracic limb, at the lateral end of the cubital crease. Find by flexing the elbow.
Bl 17	Diaphragms Transport	Located 1.5 cun lateral to the caudal border of the dorsal spinous process of the 7th thoracic vertebra.
Ki 27	Elegant Mansion	Found between the sternum and the 1st rib, 2 cun lateral to the ventral midline.

Allergic Reactions

Indicators

- Itching / Excessive scratching
- Rash
- Raised bumps
- Scabs
- Redness / Inflammation
- Loss of hair
- Blisters

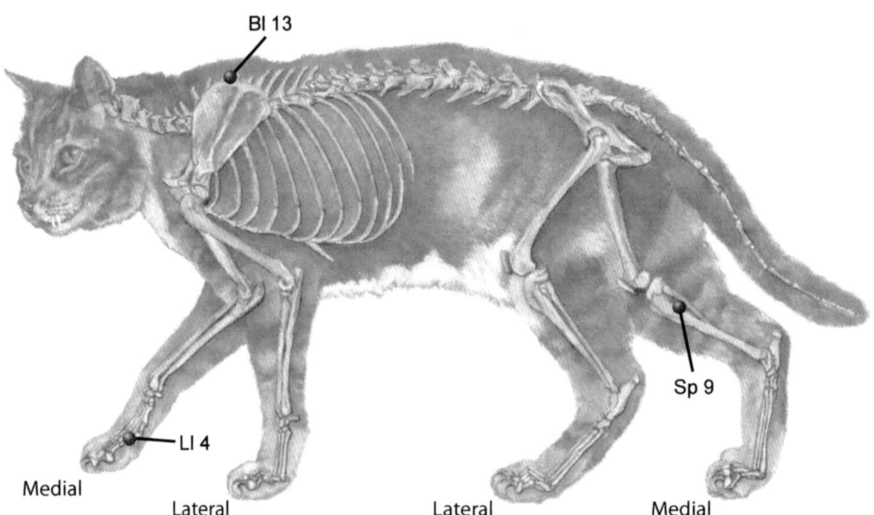

Point	Name	Location
LI 4	Adjoining Valley	Between the first (dewclaw) and 2nd metacarpal bones, on the medial side of the 2nd metacarpal.
Sp 9	Yin Mound Spring	Found on the medial side of the pelvic limb, in a depression between the caudal border of tibia and gastrocnemius muscle.
Bl 13	Lung's Transport	1.5 cun lateral to the caudal border of the dorsal spinous process of the 3rd thoracic vertebra.

Spaying / Neutering

Many good reasons for spaying your female cat or neutering your male cat exist beyond overpopulation. For example, females are less likely to develop breast cancer and will not be at risk for uterine or ovarian cancer. Males will not get testicular cancer, will be at a lower risk of transmitting diseases, and be less inclined to roam or be aggressive.

Post spaying or neutering, allow your cat to rest and recuperate as with any surgical procedure. Look for hormonal shifts that can affect the maturation process. In TCM, there will always be a level of deficiency when reproductive organs are removed. However, acupressure can help support the body's energetic ability to balance and cope with the loss.

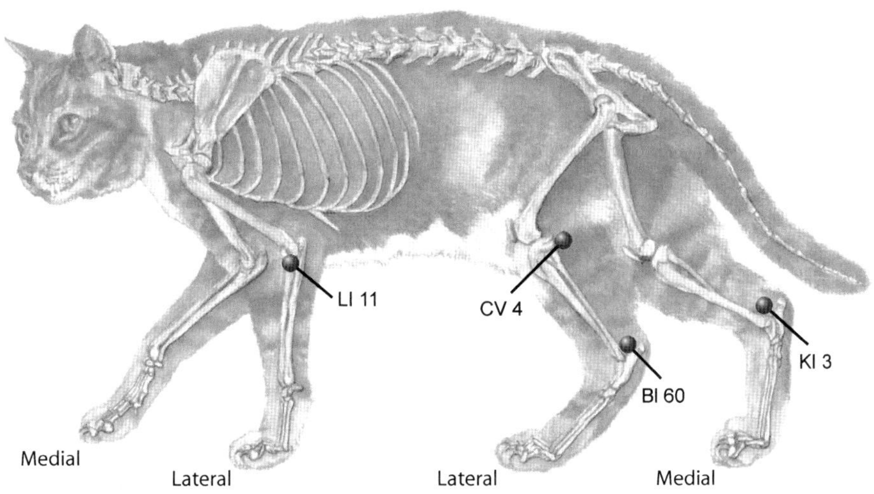

Point	Name	Location
LI 11	Crooked Pool	Found on the lateral aspect of the thoracic limb, at the lateral end of the cubital crease. Find by flexing the elbow.
Bl 60	Kunlun Mountain	Caudolateral aspect of the hind limb, at the thin fleshy tissue of the hock. Opposite Ki 3.
Ki 3	Great Stream	Found in a depression between the medial malleolus of the tibia and the calcaneal tendon. Opposite Bl 60.
CV 4	Gate to Original Chi	On ventral midline, 3 cun caudal to (behind) the umbilicus.

Trauma

Western conventional veterinary medicine is well equipped to deal with trauma and modern technology is essential when caring for your cat in a life-threatening situation. While traveling to a clinic, if you can safely work your cat's acupoints noted in the following charts, you can help mitigate the effect of the trauma. View acupressure as a support, not a substitute, for veterinary trauma care.

Remember, all emergency events require immediate veterinary attention.

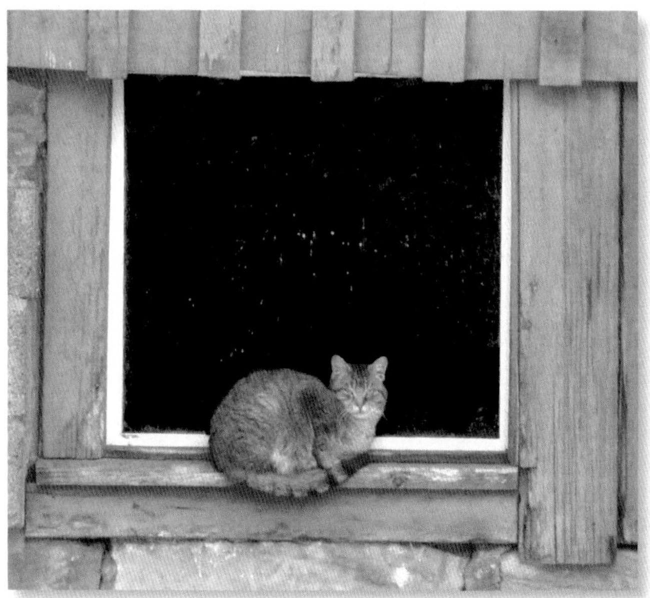

Heatstroke

Any degree of heat stroke is potentially fatal because it can damage and even shut down your cat's internal organs. Don't hesitate to get your cat to a veterinary clinic immediately. Meanwhile, you can start cooling him down by using a fan or air conditioning. Also, pouring cold running water over him can help bring his body temperature down. However, do not use ice; doing so can constrict the blood vessels and prevent body heat from escaping.

Indicators

- Elevated body temperature
- Excessive panting
- Pale gums
- Bright, dark red, or purple tongue
- Increased heart rate
- Vomiting
- Disorientation
- Unresponsive
- Collapse
- Loss of consciousness

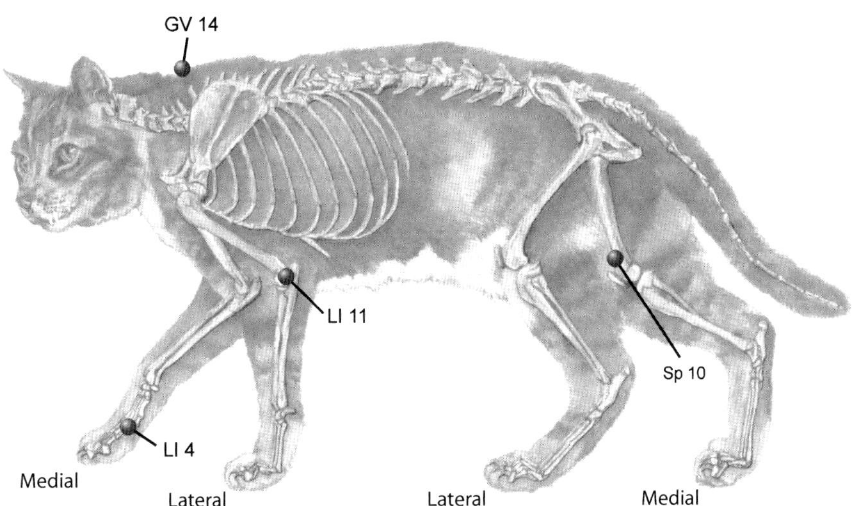

Point	Name	Location
LI 4	Adjoining Valley	Between the 1st (dewclaw) and 2nd metacarpal bones, on the medial side of the 2nd metacarpal.
LI 11	Crooked Pool	On the lateral aspect of the thoracic limb, at the lateral end of the cubital crease. Find by flexing the elbow.
Sp 10	Sea of Blood	On the medial aspect of the thigh, with flexed stifle the point is 2 cun above the patella, in a depression cranial to (in front of) the sartorius muscle.
GV 14	Big Vertebra	On the dorsal midline between the spinous processes of the last cervical and 1st thoracic vertebrae.

Shock

Shock is an acute, life-threatening condition characterized by collapse of the cardiovascular system. It requires immediate veterinary care. The points listed below are emergency points and should be used en route to the veterinary clinic.

Indicators

- Major physical injury
- Blood loss, pale gums and tongue
- Weak pulse
- Capillary refill time greater than two seconds
- Chills or shivers
- Listlessness, depressed behavior
- Rapid or shallow labored breathing
- Fixated stare with dilated pupils
- Loss of consciousness

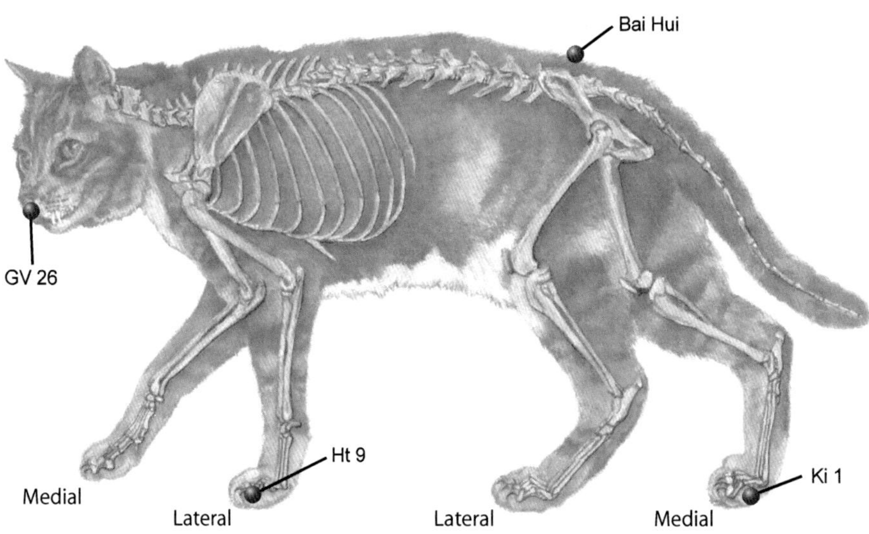

Point	Name	Location
Ht 9	Lesser Rushing	On the medial side of the 5th digit of the front paw, at the nail bed.
Ki 1	Gushing Spring	On the plantar surface of the hind paw, at the caudal edge of the metatarsal footpad.
GV 26	Middle of Man	On the vertical line on the upper lip at the level of the lower edge of the nostrils.
Bai Hui	100 Meetings	At the lumbosacral space, on the dorsal midline.

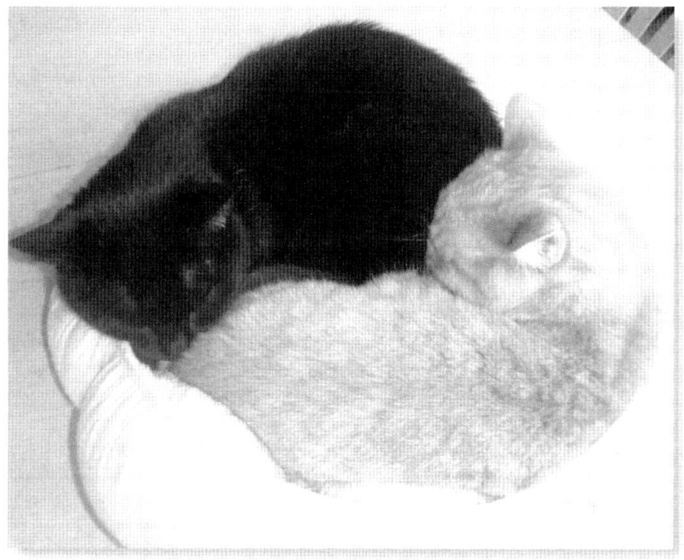

**They are not brethren, they are not underlings;
They are other nations caught with ourselves
in a net of life and time.**

— *Henry Beston*

Photographic Credits

Thank you to all the fine photographers who happily contributed the following photos of their favorite cats. We appreciate and enjoy including them in *ACU-CAT.* If we have inadvertently missed crediting your photo, our apologies, and please let us know so we can update the list.

– Thank you!

Page	**Photographer**
7	Pam Holt
9	Karen Refsnyder
13	Gabriel Alt
19, 41, 83	Kim Bauer
28, 37, 79, 86, 89, 108, 128, 131, 135, 138, 183	Sandra Osborne & MB Hall
50, 67, 85, 98, 123, 128	Kim Baker
71, 104, 150, 151, 157	Karen Tracanelli
102	Betty Gower
103, 113, 120, 127	Grant Dunmire
117	Jan Evans
143	Marc Horowitz
163	Anne-marie Hoogendijk
180	Joey Golgosky

Glossary

Abdominal cavity — The cavity of the body located between the diaphragm and the pelvis. This cavity contains the abdominal organs.

Acetabulum — The socket portion of the ball-and-socket hip joint. It is formed at the junction of the ilium, ischium and pubis bones of the pelvis. The cup-shaped socket of the hip joint that carries the head of the femur.

Accumulation Points — Specific acupressure points located on a meridian where the chi accumulates. Used primarily for acute conditions, especially if pain is present.

Acupoints — Specific acupoints located on a meridian where chi flows close to the surface of the body. Stimulation, tonification, sedation and other techniques can be employed to manipulate the chi energy of the body at these locations. There are 361 acupoints located along the 12 Major Meridians.

Acupressure — An ancient healing art that moves and balances chi and blood by use of pressure applied at specific acupoints along the meridian system. Used to release muscular pain, tension, to increase circulation and treat a variety of ailments and conditions by balancing vital substances.

Acupuncture — The manipulation of chi energy by use of needle insertions at specific acupoints along the meridian system. Used to release muscular pain, tension, to increase circulation and treat a variety of ailments and conditions by balancing vital substances.

Acute — A condition having a short and relatively sudden course, not long-term.

Alarm Points — A classification of acupoints where the chi energy of a particular organ accumulates when the organ is imbalanced. Alarm points are used in both assessment and treatment and are often used in conjunction with the Association points.

Antebrachium — The forearm region of the thoracic limb.

Glossary

Anti inflammatory An agent that relieves inflammation or swelling, and heat, of the tissues.

Anterior Situated at or directed toward the front. Situated in front of some specific reference point.

Appendicular skeleton The skeleton of the limbs.

Artery The blood vessel carrying blood away from the heart into the system. The blood vessels furnish oxygen and nutrients to the body tissues.

Articular Pertaining to a joint.

Articular surface The smooth joint surface of a bone that contacts another bone in a synovial joint.

Articulate To join or unite by joints.

Associated meridians A pair of Yin and Yang meridians. Each of the twelve major meridians has an associated meridian partner, making a total of six paired meridians. Point work on either of the paired meridians serves to balance the energy flow of the other.

Association Points A classification of points located along the inner channel of the Bladder meridian. Each of the 12 Major Meridians has a unique Association point that exhibits an internal / external relationship with each of the organs. These points can indicate a blockage in their corresponding meridian and are often used in conjunction with the Alarm points to help identify the level of organ involvement.

Asternal ribs Ribs not joined to the sternum.

Glossary

Atlas	The first cervical vertebra (C 1). It forms the atlanto-occipital joint with the occipital bone of the skull and the atlanto-axial joint with the axis C 2).
Atrophy	Decrease in size of muscle or organ resulting from lack of use or disease.
Autoimmune disease	Refers to a variety of serious, chronic illnesses where the body's immune system becomes misdirected, attacking the organs it was designed to protect.
Axis	The second cervical vertebra (C 2). It is the longest of the vertebrae in the column.
Axial skeleton	The skeleton of the head and trunk.
Belly	The thick, central portion of a muscle.
Body fluids	In TCM, the collective term for all the normal fluids of the body. These include saliva, gastric juice, intestinal juice, and the liquids of the joint cavities, as well as tears, nasal discharge, sweat, and urine.
Brachium	The upper arm, the area of the thoracic limb between the elbow and the shoulder.
Calcaneus	The irregular quadrangular bone located at the back of the hock, part of which points upward and backward to form the point of the hock.
Carpus	The segment of limb between the radius, ulna, and metacarpus, made up of seven bones. These bones are arranged in two rows, known as the wrist in cats.
Cartilage	A dense, gristly, type of connective tissue found on the articular ends of bones.

Glossary

Caudal	Situated more toward the tail than some specific reference point.
Central nervous system	The brain and spinal cord.
Cervical vertebrae	The seven bones of the neck portion of the spinal column, includes the atlas and the axis.
Channel Chi	The aspect of chi that flows through the meridian or channel system. It is the aspect of chi that is most available for adjustment or influence by acupressure or acupuncture.
Chi	Life-promoting energy present in all of nature. There are different types of chi, defined by location and function.
Chronic	A condition that persists for a long time with little change or improvement.
Claws	Accessory appendages of the integumentary system present mainly in carnivores for the purpose of grasping prey and self-defense.
Closing	The third phase of an acupressure session. The closing serves to connect the energy flow between the acupoints stimulated during the session. It also repatterns cellular memory and benefits chronic pain.
Coccygeal vertebrae	The 5th region of the vertebral column located at the tail, also known as the caudal vertebrae.
Condyle	A rounded projection on a bone, mostly for articulation with another bone.
Conception Vessel	One of the eight Extraordinary Vessels. A yin vessel running along the ventral midline.

Connecting Points A classifications of acupoints that connect the Yin and Yang energies of the sister meridians. These points help resolve blockages between the sister meridians and enhance point work.

Connective tissue A fibrous type of body tissue. This tissue supports and connects the internal organs, forms bones and the walls of blood vessels. It also attaches muscles to bones, and replaces other types of tissue after injury.

Control Cycle The sequence of the Five-Element Theory in which each element controls another and is itself controlled by another element. This sequence helps ensure balance is maintained among the five elements.

Costal arch The rim to the bony thorax formed by the conjoined asternal ribs and their connecting elastic tissue.

Costal cartilages The cartilaginous ventral portion of a rib.

Cranial Anatomical term meaning the positioning of a point or structure toward the head, the front or superior end of the body.

Creation Cycle The sequence of the Five-Element Theory in which each element creates another and is itself created by another element. This sequence helps ensure that a balance is maintained among the five elements.

Cun Translates to 'little measurement'. Used to help define a more exact location for acupressure points on the body.

Cutaneous Pertaining to the skin.

Deficiency A condition of insufficiency or too little of something.

Dewclaw A digit that does not reach the ground, such as the first digit of dogs and cats.

Glossary

Digit — A toe made up of two or three bones called phalanges.

Distal — Refers to structures or points that lie furthest away from the body or trunk. Opposite of proximal.

Distal phalanx bone — The bone of the phalanx that is located most distally from the body, the tip of the digit.

Distal points — Acupressure points located away from the area they benefit. For instance, Liv 2 is a distal point when used to strengthen the eyes.

Dorsal — An area directed toward or situated on the back surface, the surface facing away from the ground.

Endocrine system — The system of glands that controls and regulates body functions through the internal secretion of hormones, which are placed directly into the bloodstream where they act throughout the body.

Estrous — The entire reproductive cycle of the cat. Regularly occurring periods during which a female is sexually active and receptive.

Excess — A condition of surplus or too much of something.

Extension — The joint movement that increase the angle between two bones.

Extensor muscles — Any muscle that extends a joint.

External — This term refers to all that is outside the body. Located on or near the outside.

Extraordinary Vessels — Eight vessels which act as reservoirs of energy for the major meridians. They absorb energy from the major meridians or transfer energy to the major meridians as needed.

Fascia A sheet or band of fibrous connective tissue that permeates the body. A fascia is a connective tissue that surrounds muscles, groups of muscles, blood vessels, and nerves, binding those structures together. It serves as a point of attachment for many muscles.

Femorotibial joint The joint of the femur and tibia.

Femur The thigh bone, which runs from the pelvis to the stifle.

Feral An ex-domesticated cat which has reverted to being fully wild or the wild-born (never domesticated) offspring of stray cats.

Fever An abnormally high body temperature. In cats a body temperature over 102.5° F or 39.2° C.

Flexion The act of bending or the condition of being bent.

Flexor muscle Any muscle that flexes a joint.

Fibula The smaller and lateral of the two bones of the lower end of the hind limb, from stifle to hock. Does not support any appreciable weight, mainly a muscle attachment site.

Five Phases of Transformation A conceptual framework representative of the natural phases of transformation and cycles of life and seasonal/environmental changes.

Floating rib A rib whose distal extremity is unattached.

Food Chi Also known as *Gu Chi.* It is the chi obtained from food.

Foot pad The primary weight-bearing pad of each foot, the metacarpal pad of the foreleg and the metatarsal pad of the hind leg.

Glossary

Foramen A hole in a bone.

Forearm The lower foreleg, between the elbow and wrist (carpus).

Forequarters The shoulders and the anterior limbs.

Fossa A hollow or depressed area, a trench or groove like channel.

Fu organs The six Yang organs, also referred to as the hollow organs.

Gait The manner or style of locomotion. Used often to assess the soundness of an animal. Gaits include the walk, trot, amble, pace, canter, and gallop.

Gaskin The muscular portion of the hind limb located between the stifle and the hock.

Gastrointestinal Pertaining to the stomach and intestines, it can refer to the entire digestive tract.

Gliding joint A joint in which two flat, articular surfaces rock on each other. The carpus is an example of a gliding joint.

Haunch The region of the hips and buttocks.

Hindquarters The anatomical body area located behind the flanks and includes the pelvis, thighs, and hocks.

Head A spheroidal articular surface on the proximal end of a long bone. A head is present on the proximal ends of the humerus, femur and rib. The head of a bone is joined to the shaft by an area that is often narrowed, called the neck.

Hinge joint	A joint where one surface swivels around another like a door hinge. Possible movement is flexion and extension. The elbow joint is an example of a hinge joint.
Hip dysplasia	A disorder of the hip joint in which the normally tight-fitting ball-and-socket hip joint is abnormally loose. The laxity of the dysplastic joint allows the head of the femur to move in the acetabulum, resulting in damage to the joint surfaces and osteoarthritis development.
Hock joint	The tarsal joint. The area of the tarsus on the hind limb of the cat. The ankle joint.
Humero radial	Pertaining to the humerus and radius, two bones of the thoracic limb.
Influential Points	A classification of acupoints which affect a particular functional system of the body.
Ilium	The largest of the three bones of the pelvis.
Insertion	The site of attachment of a muscle to the bone it moves. When the muscle contracts, it exerts traction on its insertion site, usually producing movement of a bone or other structure.
Internal	This term refers to all that is inside the body.
Intercostal	Between the ribs.
Interdigital	Between two digits.
Intervertebral	Between two vertebrae.
Intervertebral disk	The cartilaginous disk located between the bodies of adjacent vertebrae. Acts as a shock absorber for the vertebrae.

Glossary

Jing The life essence, or material aspect of chi, a fundamental substance stored in the kidney.

Jing-Well Point A classification of acupoints located at the digits of the cat's front and hind legs. There is one Jing-Well point for each meridian. Used to balance the meridian and for other specific conditions.

Joint capsule The enclosed area of joint formed by the ligaments and lubricated by synovial fluid.

Joints The union or junction of two or more bones. Main function of a joint is to provide motion, flexibility, absorb concussion and allow for growth. Joints can be completely immovable, slightly movable (cartilaginous joints), or freely movable (synovial joints).

Jugular groove The groove or furrow on each side of the neck in which the jugular vein is located, dorsal to the trachea.

Lame An irregularity or impairment of the function of locomotion or gait.

Lateral Anatomical term for points or structures that are situated further away from the midline or median plane of the body.

Ligament A band of fibrous tissue that connects bone or cartilages or supports viscera and serves to support and strengthen joints.

Local points Acupressure points located in the area they benefit. For example, GB 1 and Bl 1 are local points for the eye.

Lumbar Pertaining to the loins, the part of the back between the thorax and pelvis.

Lumbosacral joint The junction between the last lumbar vertebrae and the sacrum.

Lung Chi Life energy, chi, which is extracted from the air.

Lymphatic system The system that collects lymph from the tissues and returns it to the general circulation.

Mandible The bone that forms the lower jaw.

Manubrium The most cranial portion of the sternum.

Master Points A classification of acupoints which affect a regional area of the body. There are 6 Master points.

Maxilla One of two identical bones that forms the upper jaw. These bones meet at the facial midline, often considered one bone.

Medial Points or structures that are situated nearer to the midline or median plane of the body.

Membrane The thin layer of tissue that covers a surface, lines a cavity or divides a space or an organ.

Meridian blockage A condition which impedes the smooth, even, and balanced flow of chi throughout the meridian system.

Meridian system The network of invisible but real channels through which the chi flows throughout the body. These channels are located just below the skin and are connected and influence each other.

Meridians Individual energy pathways, or channels, that are part of a body wide network through which chi and blood flow.

Glossary

Metacarpals The bones comprising the paw of the front limb between the carpus (wrist) and the digits (toes).

Metatarsals The bones of the pelvic limb located between the tarsus and the phalanges.

Muscle An organ made up of bundles of fiber that have the power to contract and therefore to produce movement. Muscles function to provide locomotion and support for the body. There are voluntary and involuntary muscles.

Opening The first phase of an acupressure session. The Opening introduces 'structured' touch, provides feedback to the practitioner, and is used for assessment and treatment.

Origin The more fixed end or attachment of a muscle or the end closer to the trunk. This provides stability so that the insertion of the muscle can move bones or other structures.

Original Chi The fixed amount of chi given at conception, also known as Source chi or Prenatal chi.

Palmar Refers to the back surface of the forelimb.

Palpation To examine or explore by touching usually as a "diagnostic" assessment tool.

Patella The kneecap. A large sesamoid bone at the femorotibial joint.

Pectoral Pertaining to the chest or breast area.

Pelvic limb Either hind leg.

Pelvis The bony girdle comprised of the ilium, ischium, and pubis.

Periosteum The fibrous membrane that covers the outsides of bones except for their articular surfaces.

Phalanx A bone of a digit (toe or finger).

Plantar Refers to the back surface of the hind limb.

Point of hock The summit of the calcaneus. The calcaneon tuber.

Point Work The stimulation of acupoints located along the meridian system.

Point Work Techniques The procedures used to stimulate points. There are several techniques a practitioner may use each has a unique stimulating quality.

Protective Chi The chi that protects the body from harmful external forces or pathogens.

Posterior Directed toward or situated at the back.

Proximal Refers to structures or points that lie nearest to the body or trunk.

Pubis The cranioventral part of the pelvic girdle.

Queen An unspayed female cat. Also spelled *queean*

Rostral Structures or points that are located closer to the nose. Generally used to describe positions and directions only on the head.

Glossary

Sacral vertebrae The vertebrae of the pelvic region. The are fused into a solid structure called the sacrum. The sacrum forms a joint with the ilium of the pelvis on each side called the sacroiliac joint.

Sacroiliac joint The joint between the pelvis and the sacrum that joins the pelvic limb to the axial skeleton.

Scapula The flat triangular shaped bone comprising the shoulder. In domestic animals, no bony connection exists between the scapula and the axial skeleton.

Scapulo humeral joint The articular surface between the scapula and the humerus.

Sedate To disperse or decrease.

Sesamoid bones Bones present in some tendons where they change direction markedly over joints. They act as bearings over the joint surfaces, allowing powerful muscles to move the joints without the tendons wearing out as they move over the joints.

Shen Represents the 'spirit' or consciousness aspect of the animal.

Shock A condition of acute peripheral circulatory failure due to derangement of circulatory control or loss of circulating fluid.

Skeleton The bony framework of the body. There are about 240 bones in the skeleton of a cat, depending on the number of caudal vertebrae.

Skeletal muscle Striated, voluntary muscle that enables conscious movement. The type of muscle that moves the bones of the skeleton.

Smooth muscle Nonstriated, involuntary muscle having only one nucleus. The type of muscle found in soft internal organs and structures. Not under conscious control.

Source Points A classification of points that either sedate or tonify, depending upon the need of the meridian at the time of stimulation. There is a Source point for each meridian and it is where Original, or Source chi, can be accessed.

Spinous processes The upward projections of each vertebrae.

Sternal ribs Ribs that are attached to the sternum.

Sternum A longitudinal, unpaired plate of bone forming the middle of the ventral wall of the thorax. It has three parts, the manubrium, the body and the xiphoid process.

Stifle The 'knee' on the hind leg of the cat.

Striated muscle Striated muscles are mainly attached to the skeleton. Their movements are under the conscious control of the individual,and are involved with such things as walking, eating, tail wagging, eye movement, etc.

Superficial Structures that occur near the surface of the body.

Suspensory ligaments A ligament whose function is to support or hold up a part of the body or an organ.

Synovial fluid The yellow-white transparent viscous fluid secreted by the synovial membrane and found in joint cavities, bursae and tendon sheaths. It serves to lubricate moving parts and nourish articular cartilage. Resembles egg whites.

Talus The most proximal of the tarsal bones.

Glossary

Tarsus The joint of the distal hind limb. It is composed of numerous, small short bones. The proximal border of the tarsus articulates with the tibia and fibula.

Tendons A fibrous cord which attaches muscles to bones or other structure. When the muscle contracts, the tendon is pulled. They serve to convey an action to a remote site, change the direction of pull, and focus the energy.

Thoracic cavity The chest cavity. It is separated from the abdominal cavity by the thin, sheet like diaphragm.

Thoracic limb The front limb.

Thoracic vertebrae The 2nd segment of the vertebral column, made up of 13 vertebrae. Located between the cervical and lumbar vertebrae.

Thorax The part of the body between the neck and the abdomen. The chest. Separated from the abdomen by the diaphragm, walls are formed by pairs of ribs.

Tibia The larger and inner bone of the hind limb, below the stifle. The main weight bearing bone of the lower leg.

Tibial crest A longitudinal ridge on the front of the proximal end of the tibia.

TMJ Temporomandibular joint, the hinge joint on each side of the lower jaw that connects it with the rest of the skull.

Tom A male cat, particularly an uncastrated male; also a "full tom"

Tonify To increase or strengthen.

Trochanter One of the three tuberosities on the femur. The greater trochanter is located at its upper end on the lateral surface, the lesser trochanter is located toward the upper end on its medial surface and the third trochanter is located more distally on the lateral surface.

Tuber coxae The ventral border of the iliac wing. It is the cranial and caudal ventral iliac spines and the space between them.

Tuber sacrale The most prominent medial prominence on the ilium, above the sacroiliac joint.

Tuberosity Elevations or protuberances on bones to which muscles are attached.

Ulna One of the two bones (the radius is the other) of the foreleg that form the antebrachium. The ulna forms a major portion of the elbow joint with the distal end of the humerus.

Vascular system The blood vessel network of the body.

Ventral Directed toward or situated on the belly surface toward the ground. The opposite of dorsal.

Vertebra Any of the separate segments comprising the spine. They support the body and provide the protective bony corridor through which the spinal cord passes.

Xiphoid process The pointed process of cartilage connected with the posterior end of the body of the sternum.

Zygomatic arch The bony arch below and behind the eyes of common domestic animals. In dogs and cats it forms the widest part of the skull.

Bibliography

Altman, Sheldon, DVM. *An Introduction to Acupuncture for Animals.* Chen's Corporation, Monterey Park, CA. 1981.

Beinfield, Harriet, L.Ac. & Korngold, Efrem, L. Ac., OMD. *Between Heaven and Earth, A Guide to Chinese Medicine.* Ballentine Books, New York, NY. 1991.

Birch, Stephen and Matsumoto, Kiiko, *Five Elements and Ten Stems.* Paradigm Publications, Brookline, MA. 1983.

Cohen, Misha Ruth, OMD, Lac. *The Chinese Way to Healing: Many Paths to Wholeness.* A Perigree Book, The Berkley Publishing Group, New York, NY. 1996.

Connelly, Dianne, M., Ph.D., M. Ac. *Traditional Acupuncture: The Law of the Five Elements.* The Centre for Traditional Acupuncture, Columbia, MD. 1989.

Fox, Michael W. Ph.D., D.Sc. *The Healing Touch.* New Market Press, New York, NY. 1990.

Lade, Arnie. *Acupuncture Points: Images & Functions.* Eastland Press, Inc. Seattle WA. 1989

Maoshing Ni, Ph.D. *The Yellow Emperor's Classic of Medicine;* New Translation of the Neijing Suwen with Commentary. Shambhala Publications, Inc. Boston, MA. 1995

Maciocia, Giovanni, CaC. *The Foundations of Chinese Medicine, A Comprehensive Text for Acupuncturists and Herbalist, Second Editions.* Churchill Livingstone (Elsevier Limited). 2005.

Mann, Felix, MB. *Acupuncture, The Ancient Chinese Art of Healing and How It Works Scientifically.* Vintage Books, New York, NY. 1973.

Schoen,Allen,M. *Veterinary Acupuncture, Ancient Art to Modern Medicine, Second Edition. Mosby (Elsevier affiliate).St. Louis, MO. 2001*

Schoen, Allen M., DVM, MS and Wynn, Susan, DVM. *Complimentary and Alternative Veterinary Medicine.*Mosby (*Elsevier affiliate).* 1998.

Schwartz, Cheryl, DVM. *Four Paws Five Directions, A Guide to Chinese Medicine for Cats and Dogs.* Celestial Arts, Berkeley, CA. 1996.

Bibliography

Stux, Gabriel, & Pomeranz, Bruce. *Basics of Acupuncture.* Springer-Verlag, Berlin, Heidelberg, New York. 1991.

Wiseman, Nigel, Ellis, Andrew. Fundamentals of Chinese Medicine, Revised Edition. Paradigm Publications, Brookline, Ma.1996.

Wu, Shi Cun, *Diagnostics: TCM Study Guide Series.* Kang Tai Press, Inc., Chicago. 1998

Xie, Hulsheng,CVM, ph.D., MS, Preast, DVM, Vanessa. *Traditional Chinese Veterinary Medicine,* Volume 1: Fundamental Principles. Jing Tang. 2005

Xie, Hulsheng,CVM, ph.D., MS, Preast, DVM, Vanessa. *Xie's Veterinary Acupuncture.* Blackwell Publishing. Ames, Iowa. 2007

Xinnong, Cheng. *Chinese Acupuncture and Moxibustion.* Foreign Language Press, Beijing, China. 1987

Yanchi, Liu. *The Essential Book of Traditional Chinese Medicine,* Volume 1 Theory. Columbia University Press, New York. 1988

Zhixian, Long, Editor, *Diagnostics of Traditional Chinese Medicine.* Academy Press [Xue Yuan]

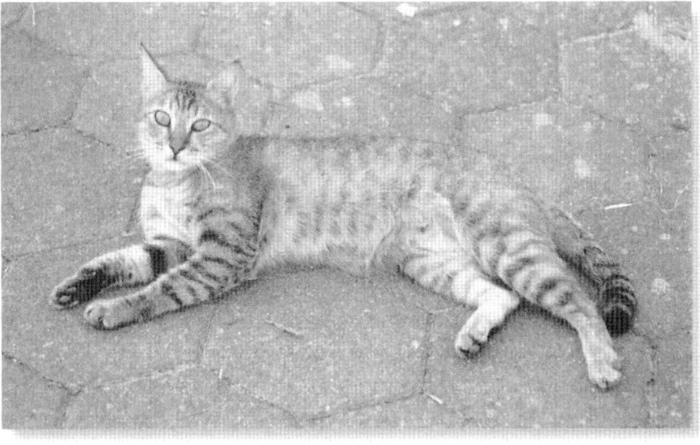

Index

A

Acupressure Session 3, 17, 29, 31, 45, 87, 89, 90, 92, 94, 98, 106, 115, 116, 117, 118, 119, 122, 129, 131, 132, 133, 135, 136, 137, 142, 146, 161, 163, 176

Aggression 152, 156

Aging 143, 144

Alarm Points 92, 93, 110, 112, 125, 127, 185

Allergies 8, 176

Anxiety 8

Arthritis 58, 98, 129, 140, 146, 163

Arthritis 146

Association Points 90, 91, 112, 124, 127

Atrophy 46, 48

B

Behavior 1, 4, 7, 8, 48, 72, 108, 109, 142, 150, 151, 153, 156

Bi Syndromes 163

Blood Deficiency 42, 176

C

Cervical 164

Compulsive Behavior 34

Conjunctivitis 175

Constipation 34, 158

Cough 157

D

Deafness 64

Defensive Chi 16, 17, 32, 161

Deficiency 176

Dental 16, 88, 96

Diarrhea 34, 157

Digestive Disorders 38, 42, 68

Distal Acupoints 141

E

Ear Problems 58, 64

Earth Element 38, 42

Edema 42, 64

Eight Principles 114

Elbow 34, 48, 61, 65, 85, 86, 88, 93

Emotional Issues 32, 34, 38, 42, 46, 48, 52, 58, 61, 64, 68, 72, 76

Essence 27, 34, 42, 58, 75, 94, 131, 143, 161

Estrous 58

Excess 21, 94, 100, 107, 131

F

Fear 52, 152, 154

Fever 169, 191

Fire Element 46, 48, 61, 64

Five-Element Theory 22, 24, 114

Four Examinations 104, 105, 109, 110, 111, 113, 118, 119, 121, 126, 139

Index

G

Gall Bladder Meridian 68

Gastrointestinal 97, 157

Governing Vessel 75, 80, 81, 82, 83, 114, 161

Grief 155

H

Health Issues 92, 104, 118, 157

Heart Chi 46

Heart Meridian 46, 47

Hip Dysplasia 166

Hock Problems 68

I

Immune System 16, 17, 161, 162, 168, 176

Immune System Chi 16, 17

Infection 172, 173

Influential Points 98, 99

Internal Pathogens 61

Itchy Skin 177

J

Jing 45, 58, 89, 100, 101, 143, 194

Jing-Well 89, 100, 101

K

Kidney Chi 58, 110, 120

Kidney Meridian 59, 60

L

Lactation 96

Lameness 166, 167

Large Intestine Meridian 35, 36

Law Of Integrity 12, 30, 104, 114

Lethargy 21, 35, 157

Liver Chi 161

Liver Meridian 72, 73, 74

Local Acupoints 141

Loss Of Consciousness 181, 182

Lower Back Soreness 52

Lung Meridian 29, 30, 32, 34, 100, 132

M

Marrow 98, 99

Master Points 96, 97

Metabolic 64

Metal Element 32

Muscles 23, 38, 42, 52, 68, 88, 109, 163

N

Neck Pain 48

Nutrient Chi 16

O

Organ Prolapse 42

Original Chi 16, 94

Index

P

Pain 38, 42, 46, 48, 58, 61, 64, 68, 76, 80, 89, 108, 109, 110, 141, 147, 158, 163, 173

Pattern Of Disharmony 21, 24, 30, 31, 114

Pericardium 27, 31, 61, 62, 63, 64, 91, 93, 96, 100, 107, 111, 114, 121, 124, 125, 126, 141

Pericardium Meridian 61

R

Reproduction 16, 58, 76

Reproductive Issues 72

Respiratory 32, 34, 80, 168, 169

S

Seizures 68, 72, 100

Sensory 32, 42, 46, 58, 172

Sensory Orifice 32, 42, 46, 58, 72

Shen 27, 46, 100, 151, 160

Shen Disturbance 46, 151

Shock 182

Shoulder 167

Sinews 72

Small Intestine Meridian 48, 49, 50

Source Points 94, 95, 130

Spleen 48

Spleen Meridian 42, 43, 44

Stifle Problems 38, 42

Stomach 23, 27, 31, 38, 39, 40, 41, 42, 48, 64, 90, 91, 92, 93, 107, 114, 123, 124, 125, 126, 127, 141, 150, 160, 161

Stomach Chi 38, 160

T

Tendons 23, 72, 97, 98, 140, 141

Theory Of Chi 15

Tmj 38, 42, 48, 96

Toxins 32, 161, 162

Traditional Chinese Medicine 4, 9, 10, 11, 12, 13, 17, 19, 21, 22, 24, 25, 28, 51, 103, 114, 136, 139

Trauma 180, 206

Triple Heater Meridian 65, 66, 67

True Chi 42

U

Urinary Tract 52

V

Vaccinations 162

Vision 68, 72

Vital Substance 26, 31

Vomiting 157, 160

Index

W

Water Element 52, 58

Wood Element 68, 72

Y

Yin-Yang Theory 17, 22, 114

Z

Zang-Fu Organs 24, 26, 27, 29, 31, 107, 111, 113

Zang-Fu Theory 24, 128, 129, 131

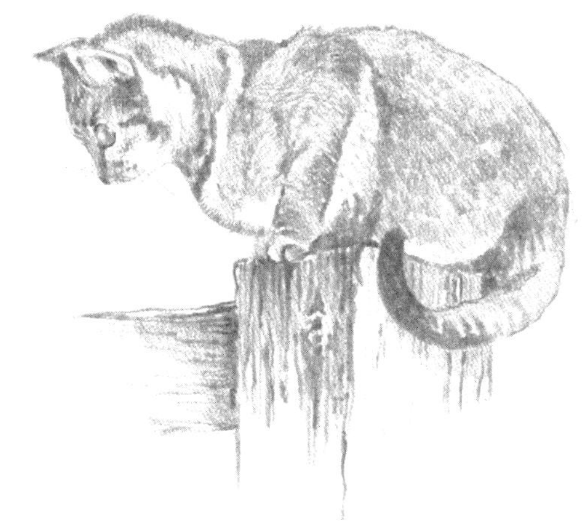

Author Profiles

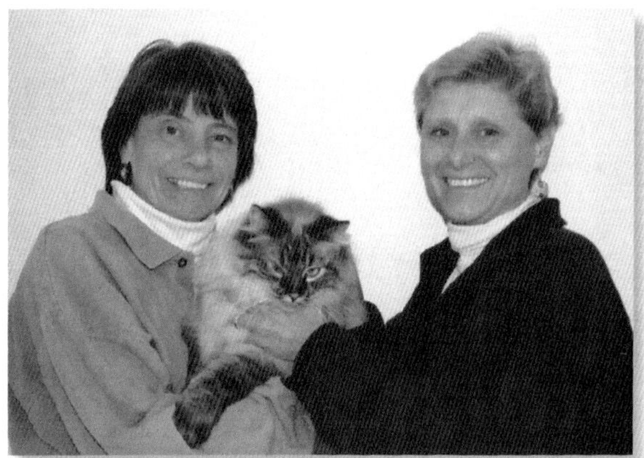

Nancy Zidonis Amy Snow

Amy Snow and Nancy Zidonis are the co-founders of Tallgrass Animal Acupressure Institute. The Institute offers hands-on and online training programs worldwide. Nancy and Amy have authored feline, canine, and equine articles for numerous publications, books, and manuals including:

ACU- CAT: A Guide to Feline Acupressure, 2nd Ed.
ACU-DOG: A Guide to Canine Acupressure
Canine Acupoint Energetics & Landmark Anatomy
Canine Health & Pathology Manual
Equine Acupoint Energetics & Landmark Anatomy
Equine Acupressure: A Working Manual
Equine Health & Pathology Manual
The Well-Connected Dog: A Guide to Canine Acupressure

Additionally, they have produced four DVDs and meridian charts for horses, dogs, and cats. Most recently, they have produced two Apps – *Equine AcuPoints* and *Canine AcuPoints*. The Apps are available at the AppStore and Google Play.

Both Nancy and Amy studied and practiced Traditional Chinese Medicine and have worked with animals for over 25 years. Their work reflects their intention of bringing animal acupressure to the people who can benefit animals most.

For more information: **www.animalacupressure.com**